T0314264

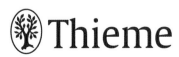

Atlas of Arthroscopic Anatomy of the Major Joints

Cristian Blanco Moreno, MD
Orthopaedic Surgeon
Hospital del Trabajador de Santiago Chile
Clinica Universidad de Los Andes
Instructor of Orthopaedics
Universidad de Los Andes
Santiago, Chile

492 illustrations

Thieme
Stuttgart · New York · Delhi · Rio de Janeiro

Library of Congress Cataloging-in-Publication Data

Names: Moreno, Cristian Blanco, author.
Title: Atlas of arthroscopic anatomy of the major joints / Cristian Blanco Moreno.
Description: Stuttgart ; New York : Thieme, [2016] | Includes index.
Identifiers: LCCN 2015040607| ISBN 9783132037915 | ISBN 9783132038011 (eISBN)
Subjects: | MESH: Arthroscopy–Atlases. | Joint Diseases–surgery–Atlases. | Joints–anatomy & histology–Atlases. | Joints–surgery–Atlases.
Classification: LCC RD686 | NLM WE 17 | DDC 617.4/720597–dc23 LC record available at http://lccn.loc.gov/2015040607

Photographer: Ana Rivero Del Rio

© 2016 by Georg Thieme Verlag KG

Thieme Publishers Stuttgart
Rüdigerstrasse 14, 70469 Stuttgart, Germany
+49 [0]711 8931 421, customerservice@thieme.de

Thieme Publishers New York
333 Seventh Avenue, New York, NY 10001 USA
+1 800 782 3488, customerservice@thieme.com

Thieme Publishers Delhi
A-12, Second Floor, Sector-2, Noida-201301
Uttar Pradesh, India
+91 120 45 566 00, customerservice@thieme.in

Thieme Publishers Rio, Thieme Publicações Ltda.
Edifício Rodolpho de Paoli, 25º andar
Av. Nilo Peçanha, 50 - Sala 2508
Rio de Janeiro 20020-906 Brasil
+55 21 3172 2297 / +55 21 3172 1896

Cover design: Thieme Publishing Group
Typesetting by DiTech Process Solutions, India
Printed in China by Everbest Printing Ltd   5 4 3 2 1

ISBN 978-3-13-203791-5

Also available as an e-book:
eISBN 978-3-13-203801-1

Important note: Medicine is an ever-changing science undergoing continual development. Research and clinical experience are continually expanding our knowledge, in particular our knowledge of proper treatment and drug therapy. Insofar as this book mentions any dosage or application, readers may rest assured that the authors, editors, and publishers have made every effort to ensure that such references are in accordance with **the state of knowledge at the time of production of the book.**

Nevertheless, this does not involve, imply, or express any guarantee or responsibility on the part of the publishers in respect to any dosage instructions and forms of applications stated in the book. **Every user is requested to examine carefully** the manufacturers' leaflets accompanying each drug and to check, if necessary in consultation with a physician or specialist, whether the dosage schedules mentioned therein or the contraindications stated by the manufacturers differ from the statements made in the present book. Such examination is particularly important with drugs that are either rarely used or have been newly released on the market. Every dosage schedule or every form of application used is entirely at the user's own risk and responsibility. The authors and publishers request every user to report to the publishers any discrepancies or inaccuracies noticed. If errors in this work are found after publication, errata will be posted at www.thieme.com on the product description page.

Some of the product names, patents, and registered designs referred to in this book are in fact registered trademarks or proprietary names even though specific reference to this fact is not always made in the text. Therefore, the appearance of a name without designation as proprietary is not to be construed as a representation by the publisher that it is in the public domain.

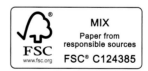

To my father, Ricardo Blanco Baeza, who passed away before this work was finished—he would be truly proud to see this book. He was an honest man with strong values who knew how to pass on those values to his loved ones and a truthful and deeply humane doctor.

To my family, Colette, Agustin, Amanda, and Antonio. Thanks for your patience and for sharing my time at home.

Contents

Preface

With the satisfaction and healthy pride of those who have traveled a long road, we present to you the first edition of the *Atlas of Arthroscopic Anatomy of the Major Joints.* As head of this project I would first like to thank God for giving us the opportunity to undertake a work of this nature and for granting us the conditions and spirit to conclude it.

All of the arthroscopic surgeons collaborating on this book were chosen because—in addition to being a reference in their relevant subspecialties—they are professionals of excellent human qualities with first-level technical and academic skills. Being able to work with a select group of specialists in arthroscopic surgery has been a privilege that has also borne the difficulty of coordinating the collaboration of doctors with tight schedules. Therefore, we appreciate their contributions to this project.

Furthermore, working with the Department of Normal Anatomy of the Universidad de Los Andes of Santiago, Chile, led by Professor Juan Carlos López, granted us sound academic support. The experience of collaborating with another field of medicine such as normal anatomy has been of great value because it is one of the most important foundations on which a surgeon has to rely in order to perform his/her procedures.

Working in the facilities of the Department of Normal Anatomy, which included the logistics for performing arthroscopic surgeries on cadavers and the subsequent dissection of each articulation, required a special coordination of support personnel, instrument technicians, and arthroscopic systems. The photographic work required extensive sessions accompanying the arthroscopies and advising on the quality of the image. Long hours were spent on text development, choosing each arthroscopic image and its relation with the external vision and real anatomy, not to mention editing each chapter with corrections following one after another. In this regard, the patient and dedicated work of the photography, editing, and graphic design team was outstanding.

We are confident that this text will be an important tool for doctors approaching arthroscopic techniques in large joints for the first time and for orthopaedic surgeons not performing these surgeries as often as in the major centers of reference. Likewise, doctors involved in teaching traumatology and orthopaedics and arthroscopic surgery will also find this book useful.

Finally, but no less important, the patient is the main focus of this effort. The motivation of this project was to be an important orientation tool for arthroscopic surgeons as per the anatomy surrounding the articulation to be treated, delivering at the same time a clear view of the relation among the important anatomical structures that may be injured during the installation of the portals. Avoiding any of these injuries or complications in a patient makes all this intellectual effort worth it. This book was designed to be timeless with solid anatomical information; therefore, we intentionally excluded clinical data.

A text of these features is not purely a technical work and does not solely depend on the specialists involved. Behind this result there was an enormous organizational work, patient coordination, a fine and accurate critical analysis, in addition to an important spiritual drive. All these roles were performed by the project director, Colette Epple, who also happens to be my wife and—thank God—continues to be after publishing this book.

Cristian Blanco Moreno, MD

Acknowledgments

Universidad de Los Andes in Santiago, Chile, and its Normal Anatomy Department

Thanks for believing in this project from the very beginning and thanks to all of the members of the Department of Normal Anatomy who shared their talents and wisdom. We appreciate the opportunity to use your excellent facilities to perform the arthroscopic procedures in the cadaveric specimens and later the dissections of the joints studied in this work. Special thanks to Marcos Valenzuela who organized the work sessions at the lab and was key during the dissections and preparation of the cadaveric specimens.

HELICO Santiago, Chile

Thanks for the logistic support during the arthroscopic procedures performed in the Department of Normal Anatomy of the Universidad de Los Andes, which required personnel and equipment and their functioning for 3 months away from their usual workplace. The cadaveric specimens, so scarce nowadays, were really an invaluable support.

Design Team

My sincere thanks to both Cristián Jiménez Riveros and Colette Epple for their careful editing of the text. Also my special thanks to the lab technician, Marcos Valenzuela Oróstica, and the lab assistant, Luis Emilio Cubillos Cornejo, who helped immensely in putting together the appropriate settings and instruments for our photographer Ana Rivero Del Rio. I am very thankful to Ana for capturing such visually engaging photographs for the book. Lastly, I would like to thank both Paula Zalazar Gaete and Paulina Vivanco Mansilla for their indispensable graphic design support and dedication to this project.

1 Shoulder

Cristian Blanco Moreno, Juan Eduardo Santorcuato Fuentes, Nelson Fritis Lama, Juan Carlos López Navarro, and Cristián Astorga Muñoz

1.1 Introduction

Shoulder arthroscopy has developed greatly over the last two decades. This technique allows a complete evaluation of the shoulder and the treatment of a variety of pathologies with minimal tissue distortion. The shoulder anatomy is complex and located near important neurovascular structures; therefore, detailed knowledge of this anatomy allows for an efficient and safe arthroscopic procedure.

The shoulder is one anatomical and biomechanical entity; however, from an arthroscopic point of view, it is easier to analyze its components separately—the glenohumeral joint, the subacromial space, and the acromioclavicular joint. This chapter presents patient positioning, external anatomical landmarks, arthroscopic portals, and the related anatomy for each of these shoulder components.

1.2 Pathologies Treated by Shoulder Arthroscopy

The therapeutic indications for a shoulder arthroscopy include:

- Rotator cuff lesions
- Labral lesions
- Glenohumeral instability
- Removal of loose bodies
- Synovium and bursa pathologies
- Septic arthritis
- Arthroscopic assistance in fracture treatment
- Acromioclavicular degenerative disease
- Acromioclavicular instability
- Subacromial pathology

1.3 External Anatomical Landmarks and Portals

To establish the shoulder portals, it is necessary to identify and mark the osseous landmarks: the acromion in its posterolateral border, the antero-distal clavicle, the acromioclavicular joint, the coracoid process, and the supraclavicular fossa (**Figs. 1.1** and **1.2**).

1.4 Patient Positioning

Shoulder arthroscopy can be performed with the patient in two basic positions: the beach chair and the lateral decubitus. In the beach chair position, the arm is located in 20 degrees of anterior flexion with the help of an assistant or an arm holder. In the lateral decubitus position, the upper limb is put in traction in 70 degrees of abduction and an anterior flexion of 20 degrees (**Fig. 1.3**). The authors of this chapter prefer the lateral decubitus position; therefore, all of the arthroscopic images included here were taken with the patient in this position. Before any arthroscopic procedure, physical examination should assess range of motion, joint stability, and laxity.

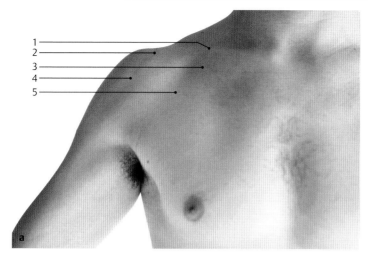

Fig. 1.1 (a, b) Anterior and posterior views of the external landmarks for a right shoulder arthroscopy.

1 Clavicle
2 Acromion
3 Coracoid process
4 Deltoid muscle
5 Deltopectoral sulcus
6 Infraspinatus muscle
7 Teres minor muscle
8 Teres major muscle
9 Triceps brachii muscle

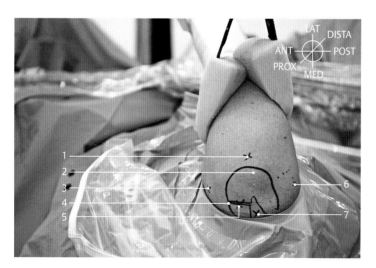

Fig. 1.2 Proximal view of a right shoulder in the lateral decubitus position showing the osseous landmarks and most frequently used portals.

1 Lateral portal
2 Acromion
3 Anterior portal
4 Acromioclavicular joint
5 Acromioclavicular portal
6 Posterior portal
7 Superior portal

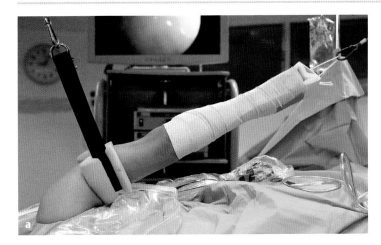

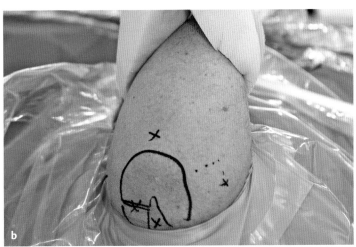

Fig. 1.3 (a, b) Patient in the lateral decubitus position for a right shoulder arthroscopy.

1.5 Suggested Arthroscopic Sequence

1.5.1 Glenohumeral Joint

Once the patient is in position, evaluate shoulder stability and range of motion. The arthroscopic evaluation of the glenohumeral joint starts from the posterior portal. The tendon of the long head of the biceps brachii muscle is the first articular structure to find and provides adequate orientation within the joint. Next, evaluate the rotator interval, the subscapularis muscle tendon, the glenoid cavity, the labrum, and the ligaments, followed by the humeral head and supraspinatus muscle tendon. Then, the arthroscope is moved posteroinferiorly to visualize the infraspinatus muscle and teres minor muscle tendons, which end at the axillary recess. Finally, the arthroscope is moved to the anterior and anterolateral portal of the glenohumeral joint as needed.

1.5.2 Subacromial Space

The subacromial evaluation should begin at the posterior portal to check the subacromial space and its bursa. Changing the orientation of the lens allows the evaluation of the rotator cuff, the acromial morphology, the coracoacromial ligament, and the inferior part of the acromioclavicular joint. The rotator cuff can be evaluated from the lateral portal of the subacromial space to better define a tear before the repair, if necessary. The anterior portal and the accessory portals (the direct acromioclavicular and superior portals) are used as needed.

1.6 Glenohumeral Joint

1.6.1 Posterior Portal

The posterior portal for the glenohumeral joint is the main portal for shoulder arthroscopy and is the first portal to be established; it is 2 cm inferior and 1 cm medial to the posterolateral corner of the acromion (**Fig. 1.4**). It allows for an initial arthroscopic evaluation and is the starting point of any procedure in the glenohumeral joint.

Anatomy and Structures at Risk

The posterior portal—when in the correct location—passes between the infraspinatus and teres minor muscles. If the posterior portal is located medially from the correct location, the circumflex scapular artery is at risk. If the posterior portal is located medially and superiorly from the correct location, the suprascapular artery is at risk. The axillary nerve and posterior circumflex humeral artery are at risk if the posterior portal is located lateral and inferior to the correct location. The anatomy of the posterior shoulder is shown in **Figs. 1.5–1.8**.

Intra-articular and Arthroscopic Anatomy

An adequate knowledge of the articular anatomy of the glenohumeral joint is key for a good arthroscopic orientation from the posterior portal and necessary to perform a safe surgical procedure. For additional safety the anterior portal is located under direct arthroscopic control from the same posterior portal (**Figs. 1.9–1.15**).

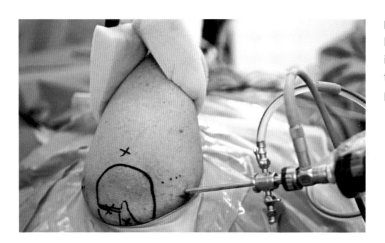

Fig. 1.4 Right shoulder in the lateral decubitus position showing the external landmarks with the arthroscope in the posterior portal.

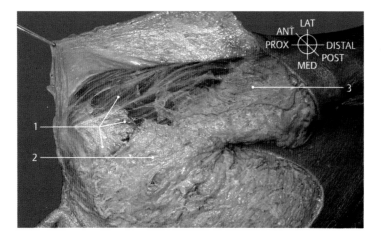

Fig. 1.5 Posterior view of a right (cadaveric) shoulder with the muscular layer partially exposed.

1 Deltoid muscle
2 Infraspinatus muscle
3 Triceps brachii muscle

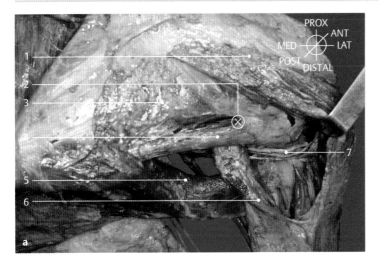

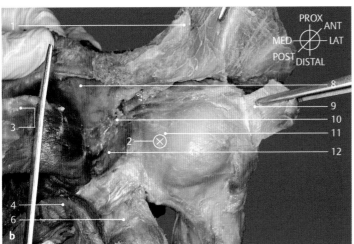

Fig. 1.6   (a, b) Posterior views of a right (cadaveric) shoulder showing the posterior muscles as well as the location of the posterior portal.

1   Deltoid muscle
2   Posterior portal
3   Infraspinatus muscle
4   Teres minor muscle
5   Teres major muscle
6   Triceps brachii muscle (long head)
7   Axillary nerve and posterior circumflex humeral artery
8   Scapula
9   Infraspinatus muscle tendon
10   Suprascapular artery
11   Posterior joint capsule
12   Circumflex scapular artery

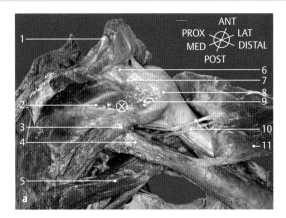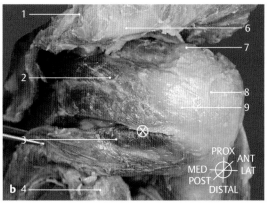

Fig. 1.7 (a, b) Posterior views of a right (cadaveric) shoulder after cutting and elevating the deltoid muscle to expose the posterior part of the rotator cuff.

1 Deltoid muscle, 2 Infraspinatus muscle, 3 Teres minor muscle, 4 Triceps brachii muscle (long head), 5 Teres major muscle, 6 Acromion, 7 Supraspinatus muscle tendon, 8 Humeral head, 9 Infraspinatus/teres minor muscle tendons, 10 Axillary nerve and posterior humeral circumflex artery, 11 Deltoid muscle cut and mobilized distally, ⊗ Posterior portal

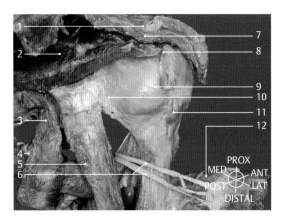

Fig. 1.8 Posterior view of a right (cadaveric) shoulder after cutting and moving the posterior muscles to expose the posterior capsule of the glenohumeral joint.

1 Deltoid muscle, 2 Infraspinatus muscle, 3 Teres minor muscle cut, 4 Teres major muscle, 5 Triceps brachii muscle (long head), 6 Axillary nerve and posterior humeral circumflex artery, 7 Acromion, 8 Infraspinatus muscle tendon cut, 9 Humeral head, 10 Shoulder joint capsule, 11 Teres minor muscle tendon cut, 12 Deltoid muscle cut and distally mobilized

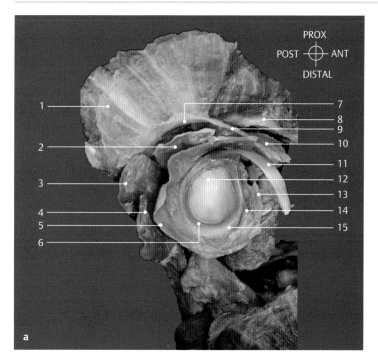

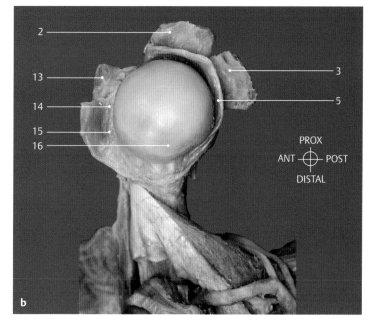

Fig. 1.9   (a, b) A right (cadaveric) shoulder that shows the lateral view of the glenoid process and the superior view of the proximal humerus.

1 Deltoid muscle
2 Supraspinatus muscle/tendon
3 Infraspinatus muscle/tendon
4 Teres minor muscle/tendon
5 Joint capsule
6 Glenoid labrum
7 Acromion
8 Clavicle
9 Coracoacromial ligament
10 Coracoid process
11 Tendon of the long head of the biceps brachii muscle
12 Glenoid cavity
13 Subscapularis muscle tendon
14 Middle glenohumeral ligament
15 Inferior synovial recess
16 Humeral head

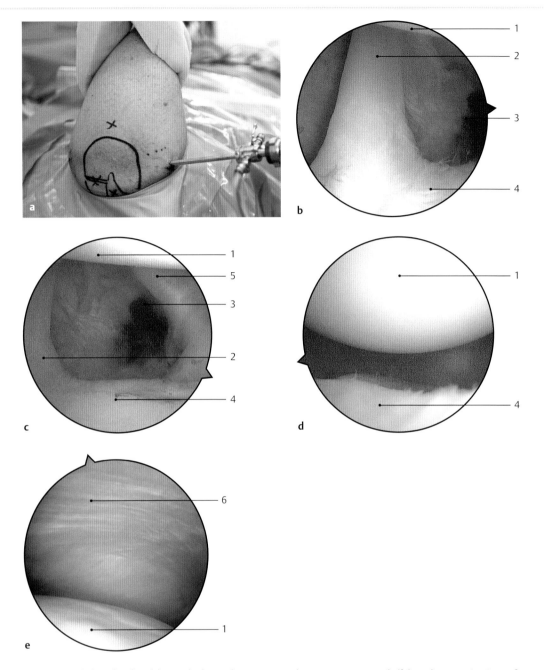

Fig. 1.10   (a) Right shoulder with the arthroscope in the posterior portal. **(b)** Arthroscopic view of the tendon of the long head of the biceps brachii muscle. **(c)** Arthroscopic view of the rotator interval. **(d)** Arthroscopic view of the humeral head and posterior labrum margin. **(e)** Arthroscopic view of the rotator cuff.

1 Humeral head, 2 Tendon of the long head of the biceps brachii muscle, 3 Rotator interval, 4 Glenoid labrum, 5 Subscapularis muscle tendon, 6 Supraspinatus muscle tendon

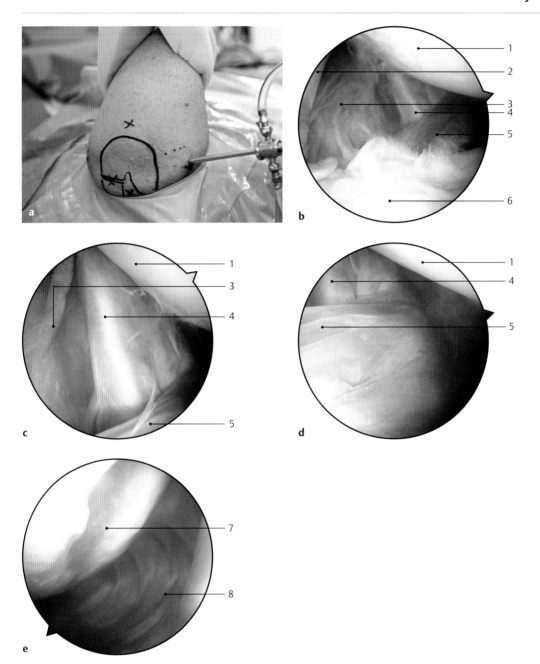

Fig. 1.11 **(a)** Right shoulder with the arthroscope in the posterior portal as the lens looks lateral.
(b) Arthroscopic view of the rotator interval. **(c)** Arthroscopic view of the subscapularis muscle tendon.
(d) Arthroscopic view of the middle glenohumeral ligament. **(e)** Arthroscopic view of the inferior joint
capsule as the lens looks medial.

1 Humeral head, 2 Tendon of the long head of the biceps brachii muscle, 3 Rotator interval,
4 Subscapularis muscle tendon, 5 Middle glenohumeral ligament, 6 Glenoid labrum (anterior),
7 Humeral head bare zone, 8 Inferior joint capsule

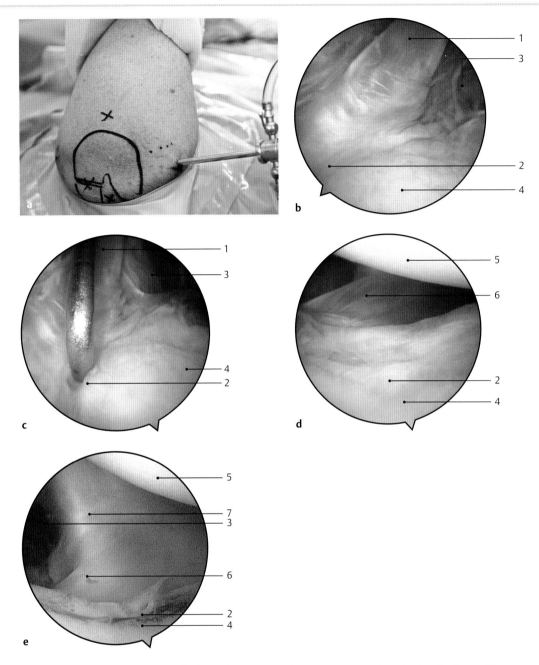

Fig. 1.12 **(a)** Right shoulder with the arthroscope in the posterior portal as the lens looks medial. **(b)** Arthroscopic view of the anterosuperior labrum. **(c)** Arthroscopic view of the palpation of the anterosuperior labrum. **(d)** Arthroscopic view of the anterior labrum and middle glenohumeral ligament. **(e)** Arthroscopic view of the anterior labrum and subscapularis muscle tendon.

1 Tendon of the long head of the biceps brachii muscle, 2 Glenoid labrum, 3 Rotator interval,
4 Articular surface of the glenoid, 5 Humeral head, 6 Middle glenohumeral ligament,
7 Subscapularis muscle tendon

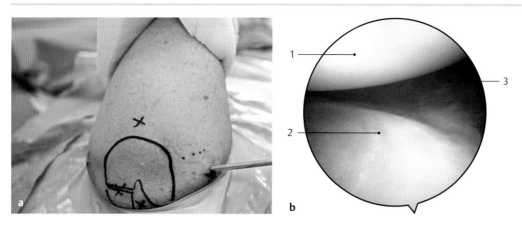

Fig. 1.13 **(a)** Right shoulder with the arthroscope in the posterior portal as the lens looks inferior. In the arthroscopic view the arthroscope then is moved back and inferiorly. **(b)** Arthroscopic view of the inferior labrum and axillary recess.

1 Humeral head, 2 Inferior glenoid labrum, 3 Articular joint capsule

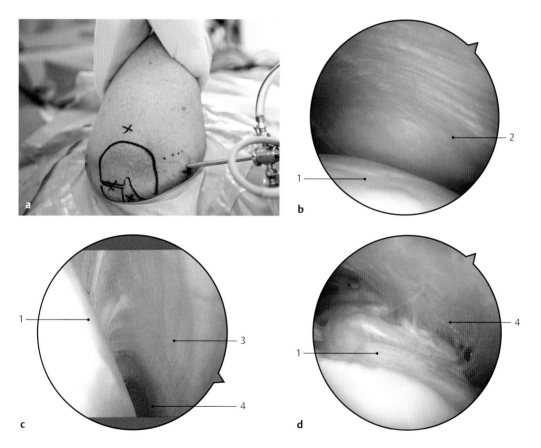

Fig. 1.14 **(a)** Right shoulder with the arthroscope in the posterior portal. The arthroscope is moved toward a superolateral position to start the evaluation of the rotator cuff. **(b)** Arthroscopic view of the supraspinatus muscle tendon. **(c)** Arthroscopic view of the infraspinatus muscle tendon. **(d)** Arthroscopic view of the teres minor muscle tendon.

1 Humeral head, 2 Supraspinatus muscle tendon, 3 Infraspinatus muscle tendon, 4 Teres minor muscle tendon

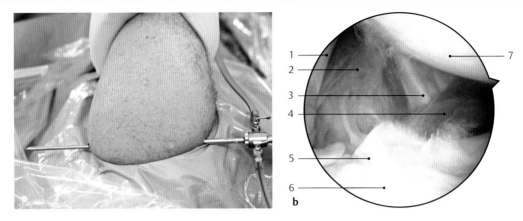

Fig. 1.15 **(a)** As the arthroscope is moved back to the starting position, a trocar is passed (with the help of the arthroscopic cannula) through the rotator interval and the skin at the location of the anterior portal. **(b)** Arthroscopic view of the rotator interval in the starting position.

1 Tendon of the long head of the biceps brachii muscle, 2 Rotator interval, 3 Subscapularis muscle tendon, 4 Middle glenohumeral ligament, 5 Glenoid labrum, 6 Glenoid cavity, 7 Humeral head

1.6.2 Anterior Portal

The anterior portal for the glenohumeral joint is 4 cm inferior to the anterior tip of the acromion and is always lateral to the coracoid process. It is used mainly as an instrumentation portal for the glenohumeral joint. The anterior portal can be performed using the outside-in technique, in a free-hand fashion with direct arthroscopic control from the posterior portal, or it can be established using the posterior portal as a reference and guide (**Fig. 1.16**).

Anatomy and Structures at Risk

The anterior anatomy of the shoulder is complex. The structures potentially at risk during anterior arthroscopic shoulder instrumentation are the cephalic vein, the lateral and medial pectoral nerves (the lateral and medial cords of the brachial plexus) and the musculocutaneous nerve, the thoracoacromial artery and its branches (clavicular, acromial, deltoid, pectoral), the axillary vein and artery, and the conjoint tendon (coracobrachialis, biceps, and pectoralis minor muscle tendons). See **Figs. 1.17** and **1.18**.

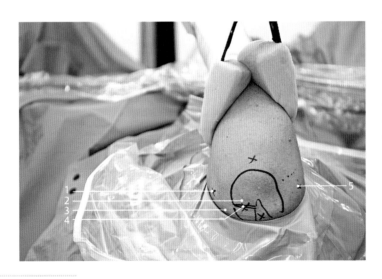

Fig. 1.16 Right shoulder showing the external landmarks for the anterior portal.

1 Anterior portal
2 Anterior tip of the acromion
3 Coracoid process
4 Acromioclavicular joint
5 Posterior portal

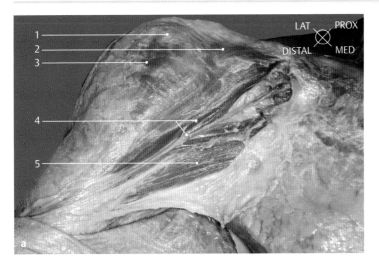

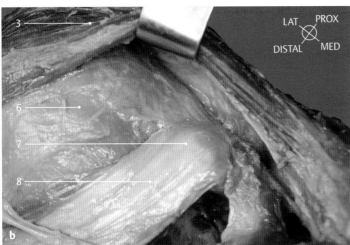

Fig. 1.17 **(a)** Anterior view of a right (cadaveric) shoulder. The dissection of the skin exposes the deltopectoral sulcus and the cephalic vein. **(b)** The deltoid muscle and cephalic vein are elevated to expose the coracoid process, the conjoint tendon, and the anterior part of the shoulder joint.

1 Anterior acromion
2 Clavicle
3 Deltoid muscle
4 Deltopectoral sulcus and cephalic vein
5 Pectoralis major muscle (clavicular part)
6 Anterior glenohumeral joint
7 Coracoid process
8 Conjoint tendon

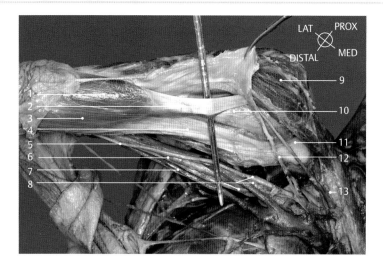

Fig. 1.18 Anterior view of a right (cadaveric) shoulder exposing the deep muscular layer of the anterior aspect of the shoulder. The pectoralis major muscle was resected and the pectoralis minor was cut at its coracoid insertion. The coracobrachialis muscle, the short head of the biceps brachii muscle (and their insertion to the coracoid process), the brachial plexus, and axillary vessels are shown.

1 Long head of the biceps brachii muscle, 2 Tendon of the long head of the biceps brachii muscle, 3 Coracobrachialis muscle, 4 Coracobrachialis tendon, 5 Musculocutaneous nerve, 6 Axillary artery, 7 Axillary vein, 8 Brachial plexus (lateral cord/posterior cord/medial cord), 9 Deltoid muscle, 10 Anterior glenohumeral joint, 11 Coracoid process and conjoint tendon, 12 Lateral pectoral nerve, 13 Clavicle

Intra-articular and Arthroscopic Anatomy

An adequate knowledge of the articular anatomy of the glenohumeral joint is important for proper orientation during arthroscopic surgery (**Figs. 1.19–1.22**). The anterior portal, as mentioned before, is used mainly as an instrumentation portal.

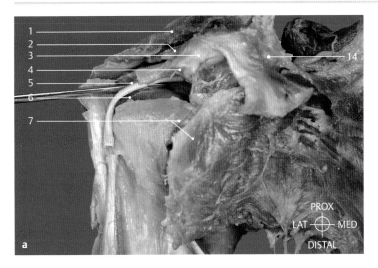

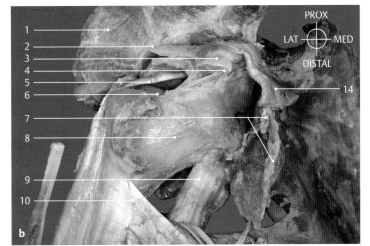

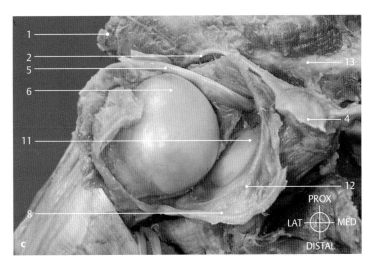

Fig. 1.19   (a) Anterior view of a right (cadaveric) shoulder.
(b) The deltoid, pectoralis major, and pectoralis minor muscles are cut and mobilized to gain access to the anterior joint capsule.
(c) Finally, the capsule is opened to expose the intra-articular structures.

1   Deltoid muscle
2   Acromion
3   Coracoid process
4   Conjoint tendon (short head of the biceps brachii muscle, coracobrachialis and pectoralis minor muscle)
5   Tendon of the long head of the biceps brachii muscle
6   Humeral head
7   Subscapularis muscle/tendon
8   Anterior joint capsule
9   Triceps brachii muscle (long head)
10   Latissimus dorsi muscle tendon
11   Glenoid cavity
12   Middle glenohumeral ligament
13   Clavicle
14   Pectoralis minor muscle tendon

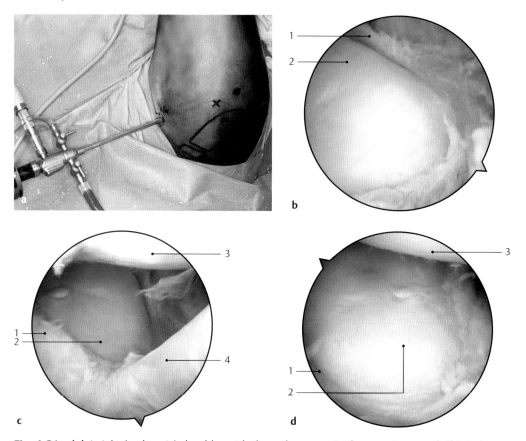

Fig. 1.20   (a, b) Arthroscopic view of a right (cadaveric) shoulder taken from the posterior portal showing the rotator interval—the spot for the anterior portal. The extra-articular view of the same right shoulder (cadaveric) shows the inside-out technique for establishing the anterior portal: a trocar is passed through the arthroscopic cannula inside the posterior portal.

1 Anterior portal, 2 Anterior tip of the acromion, 3 Acromioclavicular joint, 4 Humeral head,
5 Long head of the biceps brachii muscle tendon, 6 Rotator interval, 7 Middle glenohumeral ligament,
8 Subscapularis muscle tendon

Fig. 1.21   (a) A right (cadaveric) shoulder with the arthroscope in the anterior portal. **(b)** Arthroscopic view as the lens looks proximal. **(c)** Arthroscopic view as the lens looks proximal. **(d)** Arthroscopic view as the lens looks distal.

1 Glenoid labrum, 2 Glenoid cavity, 3 Humeral head, 4 Tendon of the long head of the biceps brachii muscle

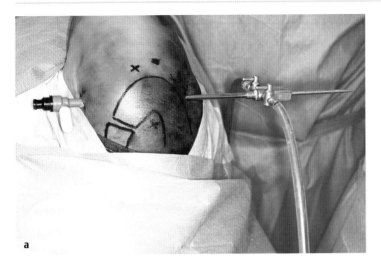

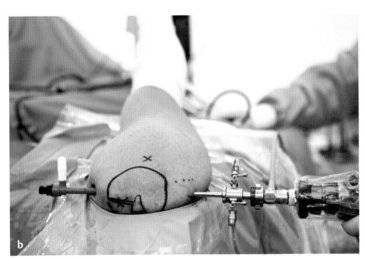

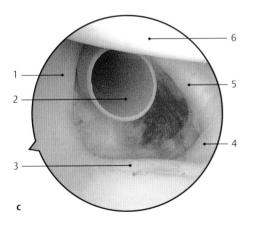

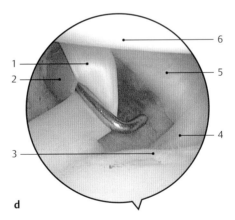

Fig. 1.22 **(a, b)** Views of a right shoulder with the arthroscope relocated in the posterior portal and the working cannula in the anterior portal. The lens looks proximal. **(c)** Arthroscopic view from the posterior portal of the rotator interval. **(d)** Arthroscopic view from the posterior portal of the tendon of the long head of the biceps brachii muscle.

1 Tendon of the long head of the biceps brachii muscle
2 Cannula in the rotator interval
3 Glenoid labrum
4 Middle glenohumeral ligament
5 Subscapularis muscle tendon
6 Humeral head

1.6.3 Anterolateral Portal

The anterolateral portal is 2 cm distal to the anterolateral border of the acromion and mainly used as a visualization portal for the instrumentation of the anteroinferior and/or posteroinferior labrum in shoulder instabilities. See **Fig. 1.23**.

Anatomy and Structures at Risk

The anterolateral portal in the glenohumeral joint is related to the musculotendinous structures of the anterior shoulder (**Figs. 1.24–1.35**).

Arthroscopic Anatomy

Arthroscopic views of the glenohumeral joint of a right shoulder from the anterolateral portal are shown in **Figs. 1.25–1.27**.

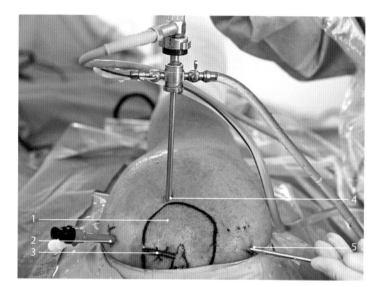

Fig. 1.23 Right shoulder with the arthroscope in the anterolateral portal.

1 Acromion
2 Anterior portal
3 Acromioclavicular joint
4 Anterolateral portal
5 Posterior portal

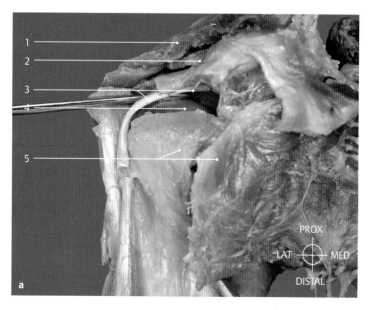

Fig. 1.24 **(a–c)** These anatomical images of a right (cadaveric) shoulder show the structures related to the anterolateral portal and the intra-articular anatomy to be evaluated through this portal.

1 Deltoid muscle
2 Acromion
3 Tendon of the long head of the biceps brachii muscle
4 Humeral head
5 Subscapularis muscle and tendon

(Continued)

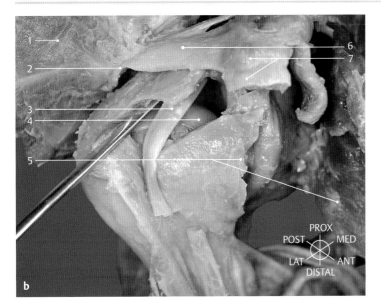

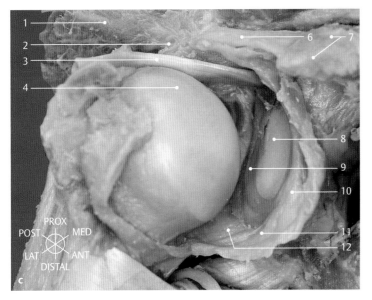

Fig.   1.24 (*continued*) **(a–c)**

1   Deltoid muscle
2   Acromion
3   Tendon of the long head of the biceps brachii muscle
4   Humeral head
5   Subscapularis muscle and tendon
6   Coracoacromial ligament
7   Coracoid process and conjoint tendon
8   Glenoid cavity
9   Glenoid labrum
10 Middle glenohumeral ligament
11 Inferior glenohumeral ligament
12 Inferior joint capsule/axillary recess

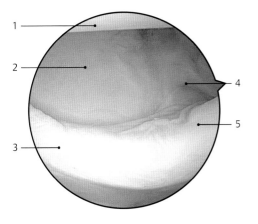

Fig. 1.25   Arthroscopic view as the lens looks proximal.

1   Humeral head
2   Glenoid cavity
3   Anterior labrum
4   Superior labrum
5   Tendon of the long head of the biceps brachii muscle
6   Inferior labrum

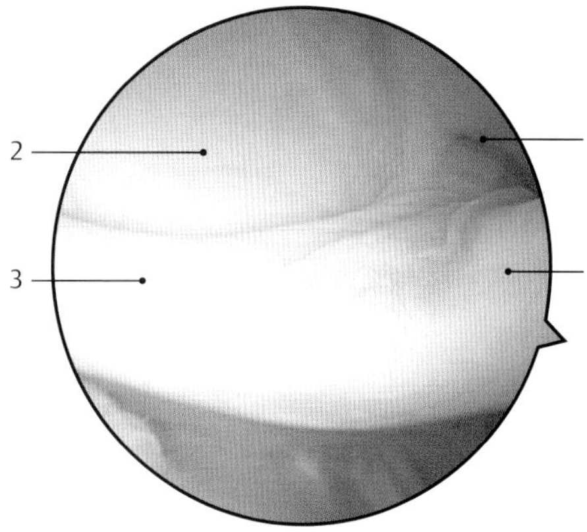

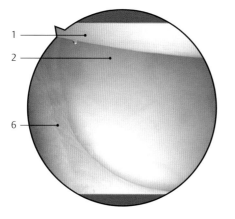

Fig. 1.26 Arthroscopic view as the lens looks proximal and anterior.

1 Humeral head
2 Glenoid cavity
3 Anterior labrum
4 Superior labrum
5 Tendon of the long head of the biceps brachii muscle
6 Inferior labrum

Fig. 1.27 Arthroscopic view as the lens looks distal.

1 Humeral head
2 Glenoid cavity
3 Anterior labrum
4 Superior labrum
5 Tendon of the long head of the biceps brachii muscle
6 Inferior labrum

1.7 Subacromial Space

The same skin incision is used for the posterior portal in the subacromial space as is used for the posterior glenohumeral portal. The arthroscope should be mobilized through the intermuscular space toward the subacromial space 1 cm proximal. Passing the trocar in between the muscles, the posterior edge of the acromion is palpable and the trocar is moved forward under its inferior surface.

The anterior portal is found under the acromion and coracoacromial ligaments. The correct location for the portal is established when the trocar inside the arthroscopic cannula hits the skin (inside-out technique). See **Fig. 1.28**.

The lateral portal can be located under direct arthroscopic control from the posterior portal (**Fig. 1.29 a, b**). This portal is key for the instrumentation in the subacromial space—first as an evaluation portal for the rotator cuff and later as a working portal (**Fig. 1.29 c**).

The anatomical landmarks and the related anatomical structures are the same as for the glenohumeral joint. The subacromial space is surrounded by osseous, muscular, and tendinous structures (**Fig. 1.30**).

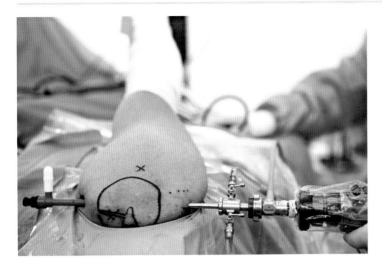

Fig. 1.28 Right shoulder showing the posterior and anterior portals for the subacromial space.

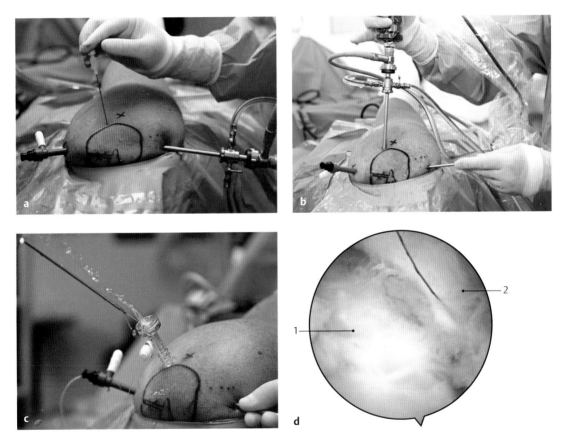

Fig. 1.29 **(a, b)** Right shoulder with the lateral portal for the subacromial space established under direct arthroscopic control from the posterior portal. **(c)** The working cannula is located in the lateral portal for the subacromial space. **(d)** Arthroscopic view from the posterior portal shows the subacromial space, and rotator cuff and working cannula in the lateral portal.

1 Rotator cuff, 2 Cannula

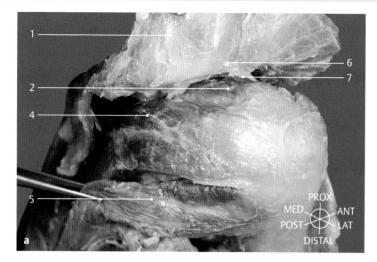

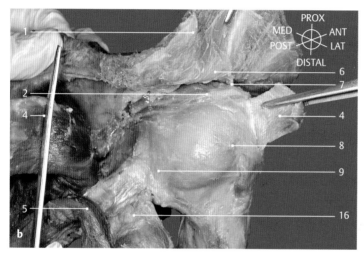

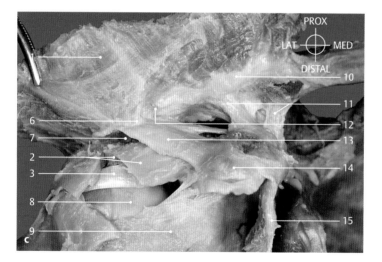

Fig. 1.30 (a, b) Posterior views of a right (cadaveric) shoulder showing the subacromial space and the surrounding anatomical structures. **(c)** An anterior view of a right (cadaveric) shoulder showing the subacromial space and the surrounding anatomical structures.

1 Deltoid muscle
2 Supraspinatus muscle/tendon
3 Tendon of the long head of the biceps brachii muscle
4 Infraspinatus muscle/tendon
5 Teres minor muscle/tendon
6 Acromion
7 Subacromial space
8 Humeral head
9 Shoulder joint capsule
10 Clavicle
11 Coracoclavicular ligaments
12 Acromioclavicular joint
13 Coracoacromial ligament
14 Coracoid process
15 Subscapularis muscle/tendon
16 Triceps brachii muscle (long head)

1.8   Acromioclavicular Joint

The direct acromioclavicular portal is located at the acromioclavicular joint line, half way between its anterior and posterior borders. The position is marked with a spinal needle to help locate the acromioclavicular joint from inside the subacromial space. The direct acromioclavicular portal is not an intra-articular evaluation portal, but instead a working portal for the resection of the distal clavicle (**Figs. 1.31** and **1.32**).

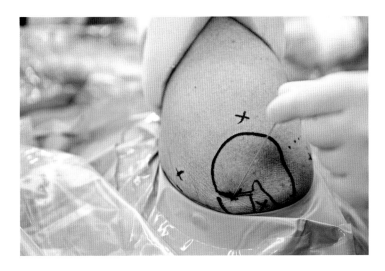

Fig. 1.31   Right shoulder showing the location of the direct acromioclavicular portal (marked with a needle).

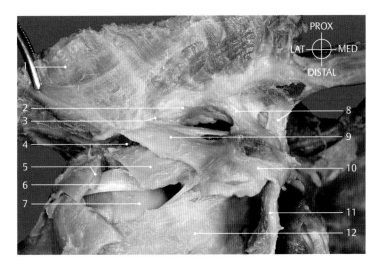

Fig. 1.32   Anterior view of a right (cadaveric) shoulder showing the anatomical structures around the acromioclavicular joint.

1 Deltoid muscle
2 Clavicle
3 Acromioclavicular joint
4 Subacromial space
5 Supraspinatus muscle/tendon
6 Tendon of the long head of the biceps brachii muscle
7 Humeral head
8 Coracoclavicular ligaments
9 Coracoacromial ligament
10 Coracoid process
11 Subscapularis muscle/tendon
12 Shoulder joint capsule

1.9 Superior Portal (Supraclavicular or Suprascapular)

The superior portal is located 1 cm in front of the spine of the scapula, 2 cm medial to the medial border of the acromion at its anterior portion, and goes through the trapezius and the supraspinatus muscles (never the tendon). This portal is used in the evaluation and the release of the suprascapular nerve at the level of the suprascapular notch. The nerve and the suprascapular artery are 3 cm away from the portal at its nearest point (**Figs. 1.33–1.35**).

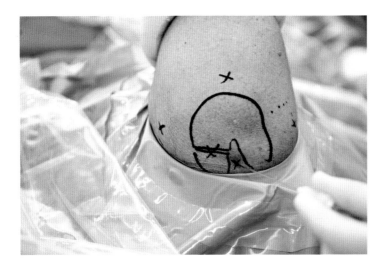

Fig. 1.33 Right shoulder showing the location of the superior portal.

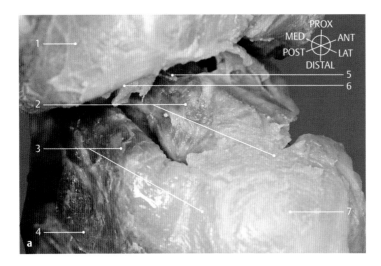

Fig. 1.34 **(a)** Right (cadaveric) shoulder with an upper view of the supraspinatus muscle belly with the deltoid muscle still attached to the acromion but mobilized.

1 Deltoid muscle
2 Supraspinatus muscle/tendon
3 Infraspinatus muscle/tendon
4 Teres minor muscle/tendon
5 Subacromial space
6 Acromion
7 Humeral head

(Continued)

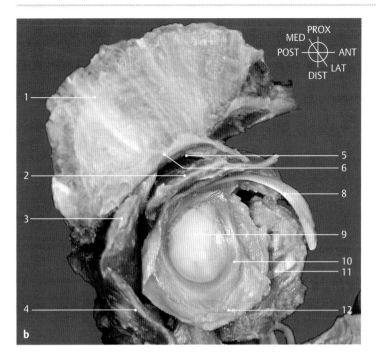

Fig. 1.34 (*continued*)
(b) A lateral view of the glenoid cavity, and the muscles and tendons related to the superior portal on its way to the supras-capular notch.

1 Deltoid muscle
2 Supraspinatus muscle/tendon
3 Infraspinatus muscle/tendon
4 Teres minor muscle/tendon
5 Subacromial space
6 Acromion
7 Humeral head
8 Tendon of the long head of the biceps brachii muscle
9 Glenoid cavity
10 Glenoid labrum
11 Subscapularis muscle tendon
12 Shoulder joint capsule

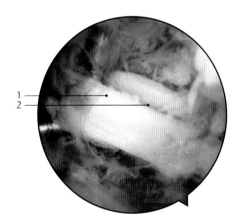

Fig. 1.35 Arthroscopic view of a right shoulder from the superior portal to evaluate the supras-capular nerve.

1 Suprascapular nerve
2 Suprascapular artery

2 Elbow

Cristian Blanco Moreno, Claudio Moraga Huerta, Juan Eduardo Santorcuato Fuentes, Juan Carlos López Navarro, and Cristián Astorga Muñoz

2.1 Introduction

Elbow arthroscopy is a technique that has become progressively safer and more effective in the treatment of the different pathologies of this joint. However, the greatest risk is possible damage to neurologic structures. Knowledge of the anatomy of the elbow region is key to avoid damage to the structures at risk during this procedure.

The objective of this chapter is to show the patient positioning, the portals needed to perform a standard diagnostic examination and therapeutic arthroscopy of the elbow, as well as the related anatomy and the structures at risk during the procedure. The anterior and posterior arthroscopic compartments and the posterolateral recess are also described.

2.2 Elbow Anatomy

The elbow joint is a triple synovial joint with two ranges of motion—flexion and extension—and those of the forearm are pronation and supination. It is composed by the articular surfaces of the humeral condyle, ulna, and the radial head.

The humeral condyle articulates with both the radius and the ulna by its two terminal articular surfaces: trochlea and capitulum, both located ~2 cm distal to the interepicondylar axis. Hence, the elbow includes three joints: the ulnohumeral joint (between the trochlear notch of the ulna and humeral trochlea), the humeroradial joint (between the radial head and the humeral capitulum), and the proximal radioulnar joint (between the radial head and the radial notch of the ulna) (**Figs. 2.1** and **2.2**).

2.2.1 Anterior Compartment of the Elbow: Cubital Fossa

The cubital fossa forms a triangular zone at the anterior and central aspect of the proximal forearm. Its cutaneous innervation is supplied mainly by the medial and lateral antebrachial cutaneous nerves, branches of the medial fasciculus of the brachial plexus, and the musculocutaneous nerve, respectively.

The interepicondylar line represents its proximal limit. The lateral margin of the pronator teres muscle and the medial edge of brachioradialis muscle correspond to its medial and lateral limits, respectively. The deep fascia of the forearm and the bicipital aponeurosis medially form its roof.

The median cubital vein lies superficial to this deep fascia and the medial antebrachial nerve crosses it. The brachialis and supinator muscle form its floor.

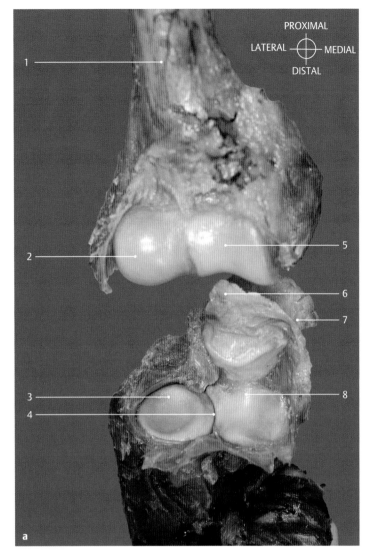

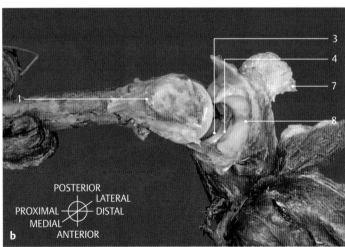

Fig. 2.1   (a, b) A right (cadaveric) elbow shows the osseous and articular structures (anterior and medial views).

1 Humerus
2 Capitulum
3 Radial head
4 Proximal radioulnar joint
5 Trochlea of the humerus
6 Posterior joint capsule
7 Triceps muscle tendon
8 Trochlear notch

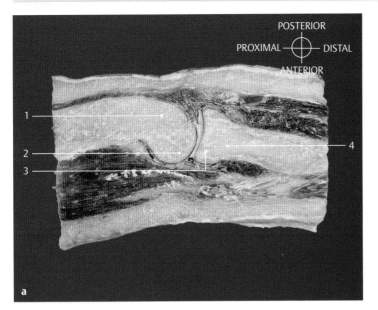

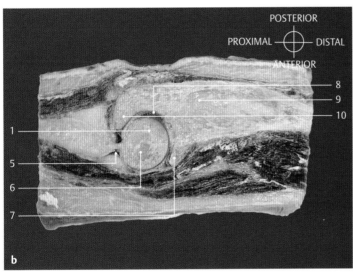

Fig. 2.2   Sagittal cuts of a right (cadaveric) elbow showing the **(a)** humeroradial and **(b)** humeroulnar joints.

1 Distal humerus
2 Capitulum
3 Radial head
4 Proximal radius
5 Coronoid fossa
6 Trochlea of the humerus
7 Coronoid process
8 Trochlear notch
9 Proximal ulna
10 Olecranon

From medial to lateral, the fossa contains the median nerve, the terminal part of the brachial artery and accompanying veins, and the initial parts of the radial and ulnar arteries. The biceps tendon and the radial nerve are just under the brachio-radialis muscle. The musculocutaneous nerve lies on the lateral margin of the biceps tendon, and it continues as the lateral antebrachial cutaneous nerve (**Figs. 2.3–2.7**).

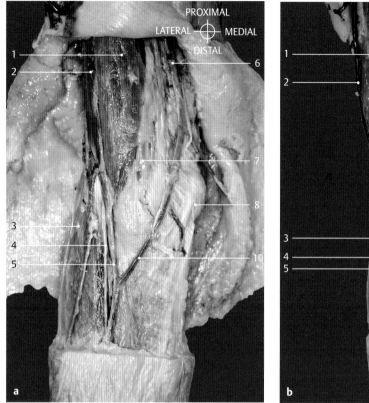
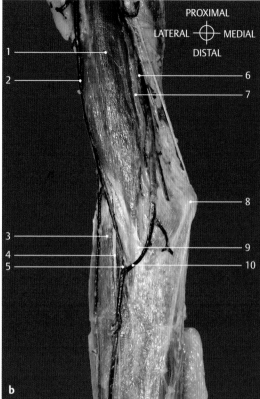

Fig. 2.3   (a, b) Anterior view of a right (cadaveric) elbow shows some of the superficial structures, especially the venous network.

 1 Biceps muscle
 2 Cephalic vein
 3 Brachioradialis muscle
 4 Lateral antebrachial cutaneous nerve
 5 Median cephalic vein
 6 Basilic vein
 7 Brachial artery
 8 Medial epicondyle
 9 Biceps muscle tendon
10 Median basilic vein

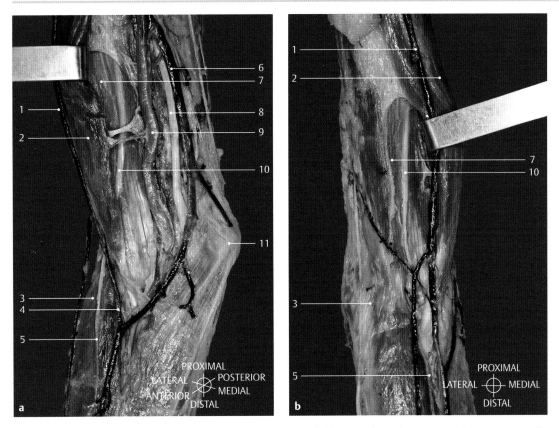

Fig. 2.4   A right (cadaveric) elbow shows the **(a)** medial and **(b)** anterolateral neurovascular structures of the distal arm on their way to the elbow region.

1 Cephalic vein
2 Biceps muscle
3 Brachioradialis muscle
4 Median cephalic vein
5 Lateral antebrachial cutaneous nerve
6 Basilic vein
7 Brachialis muscle
8 Median nerve
9 Brachial artery
10 Musculocutaneous nerve
11 Medial epicondyle

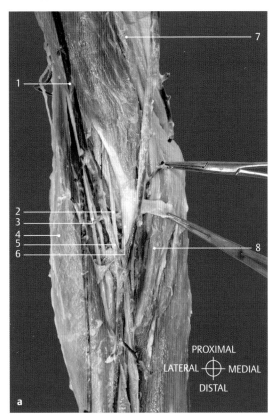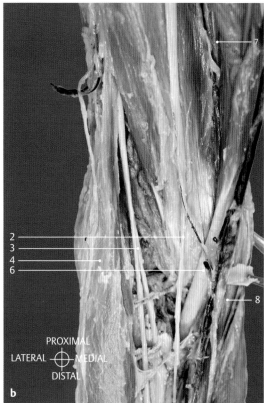

Fig. 2.5   (a, b) A right (cadaveric) elbow shows the lateral structures of the cubital fossa.

1 Cephalic vein
2 Lateral antebrachial cutaneous nerve
3 Radial nerve
4 Brachioradialis muscle
5 Median cephalic vein
6 Biceps muscle tendon
7 Brachial artery
8 Pronator teres muscle

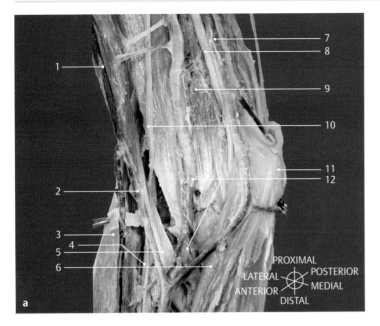

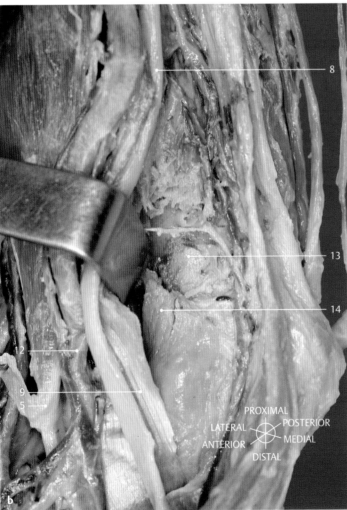

Fig. 2.6   (a, b) A right (cadaveric) elbow shows the medial structures of the cubital fossa and the joint capsule.

1 Cephalic vein
2 Median cephalic vein
3 Brachioradialis muscle
4 Radial nerve
5 Biceps muscle tendon
6 Pronator teres muscle
7 Basilic vein
8 Median nerve
9 Brachialis muscle
10 Musculocutaneous nerve
11 Medial epicondyle
12 Brachial artery (origin of the radial and ulnar arteries) and veins
13 Humerus
14 Joint capsule

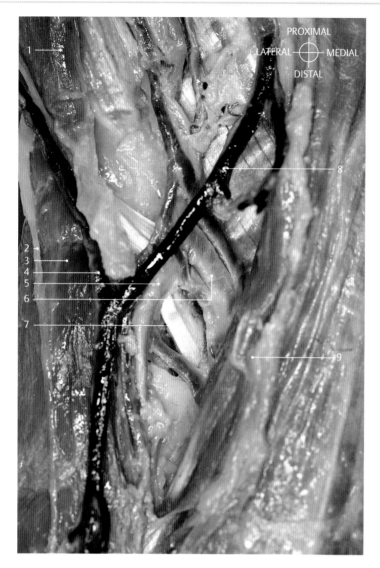

Fig. 2.7 A right (cadaveric) elbow shows the cubital fossa and the origin of the radial and ulnar arteries.

1 Biceps muscle
2 Lateral antebrachial cutaneous nerve
3 Brachioradialis muscle
4 Median cephalic vein
5 Radial artery
6 Ulnar artery
7 Biceps muscle tendon
8 Median basilic vein
9 Pronator teres muscle

2.2.2 Posterior Compartment and Posterolateral Recess of the Elbow

The posterior skin innervation is supplied by the cutaneous branches of the radial nerve, the inferior lateral cutaneous nerve of the arm, and the posterior antebrachial cutaneous nerve.

The ulnar nerve does not have branches in the arm; it runs distally and pierces the medial intermuscular septum, bending medially as it descends anterior to the medial head of the triceps muscle to the interval between the medial epicondyle and olecranon.

The posterior joint capsule is thin and in close relation to the triceps muscle tendon and anconeus muscle (**Figs. 2.8–2.10**).

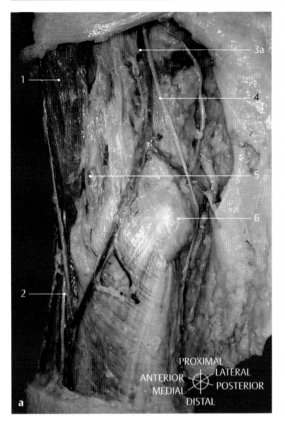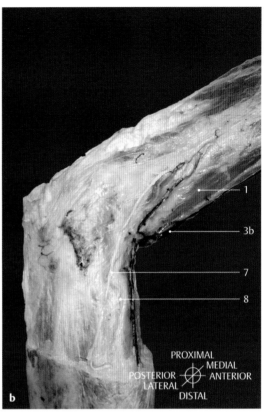

Fig. 2.8 A right (cadaveric) elbow shows part of the superficial innervation of the **(a)** posteromedial and **(b)** posterolateral aspects of the elbow.

1 Biceps muscle
2 Lateral antebrachial cutaneous nerve
3a Basilic vein
3b Cephalic vein
4 Medial antebrachial cutaneous nerve
5 Brachial artery
6 Medial epicondyle
7 Inferior lateral cutaneous nerve
8 Brachioradialis muscle

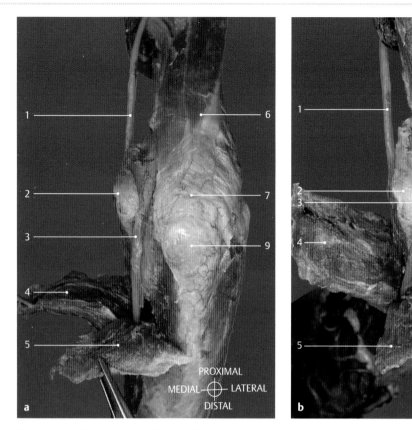

Fig. 2.9   (a, b) A right (cadaveric) elbow shows the posteromedial and posterior structures.

1 Median nerve
2 Medial epicondyle
3 Ulnar nerve
4 Flexor digitorum superficialis muscle
5 Flexor carpi ulnaris muscle
6 Triceps brachii muscle
7 Triceps brachii muscle tendon
8 Posterior joint capsule
9 Olecranon

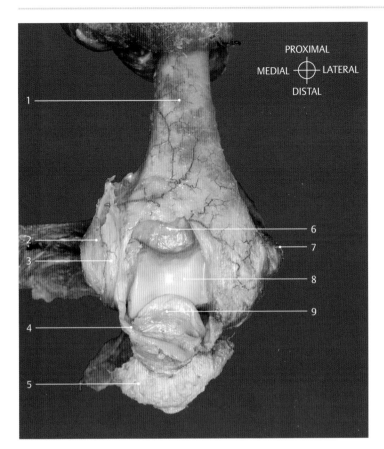

PROXIMAL

MEDIAL — LATERAL

DISTAL

Fig. 2.10   Posterosuperior view of a right elbow in a position that is similar to an arthroscopic situation (lateral decubitus). Additionally, the posterior joint capsule is opened to show the olecranon fossa.

1 Distal humerus
2 Medial epicondyle
3 Ulnar nerve (cut)
4 Joint capsule
5 Triceps brachii muscle tendon
6 Olecranon fossa
7 Lateral epicondyle
8 Trochlea of the humerus
9 Olecranon

2.3   General Indications for an Elbow Arthroscopy

The therapeutic indications for an elbow arthroscopy include:

- Articular loose bodies
- Elbow arthrosis
- Posttraumatic arthrosis
- Inflammatory arthritis
- Synovial pathology

There are some contraindications for an elbow arthroscopy. One absolute contraindication is severe anatomy distortion (soft tissue or bony structures). Another is massive heterotopic ossifications with severe extracapsular contractures. A relative contraindication is a previous subcutaneous or submuscular ulnar nerve transposi-

tion (preoperative ultrasonography is advised in these cases).

2.4   External Anatomical Landmarks

During an elbow arthroscopy the exact comprehension of the anatomy and the related neurovascular structures is the key. The osseous landmarks are subcutaneous structures and easily palpable. They are the medial epicondyle, the olecranon, the lateral epicondyle, the radial head, and the capitulum. Additionally, the ulnar nerve should be added to the list of main external landmarks. All of these structures should be marked before the elbow joint is distended with saline solution (**Fig. 2.11**).

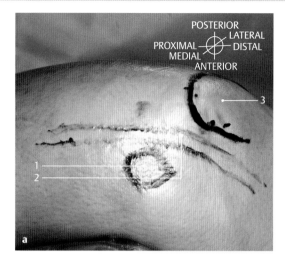
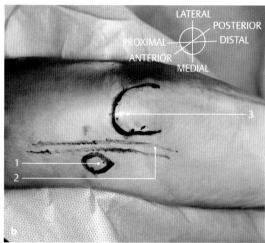
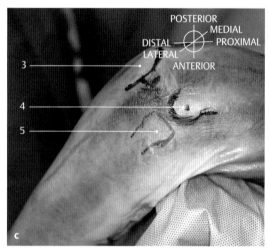
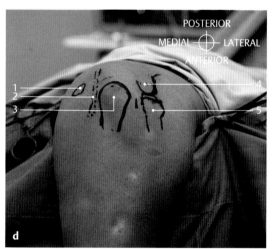

Fig. 2.11 **(a)** Medial, **(b)** posterior, **(c)** lateral, and **(d)** distal views of a right elbow (in the lateral decubitus position) with the key external landmarks marked.

1 Medial epicondyle, 2 Ulnar nerve, 3 Olecranon, 4 Capitulum/lateral epicondyle, 5 Radial head

2.5 Patient Positioning

There are four different ways to position a patient for an elbow arthroscopy: supine, supine with traction, prone, and lateral decubitus. The authors use the lateral decubitus position, as it has the advantage of more stability of the upper limb; therefore, all of the images presented are taken in this position. The lateral decubitus position allows for free flexion and extension and a comfortable approach to the anterior and posterior compartment without compromising access to the airway. Nonetheless, this setting has more restricted access to the medial zone of the elbow (**Fig. 2.12**).

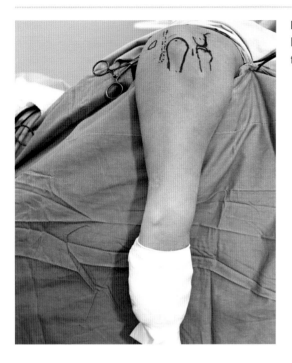

Fig. 2.12 Lateral decubitus position using an arm holder system that is fixed to the table. The elbow is the highest point of the surgical setting.

2.6   Portals

The first portal to perform depends mainly on the pathology to be treated and its location in the different elbow compartments. The classic portals for an elbow arthroscopy are the proximal anteromedial, the proximal anterolateral, the posterocentral, the posterolateral, and the direct posterolateral or "soft spot" (**Fig. 2.13**).

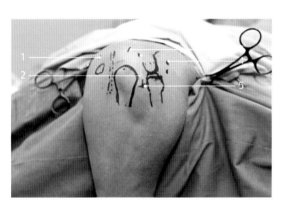

Fig. 2.13 Right elbow in the lateral decubitus arthroscopic position showing the anatomical landmarks and portals.

1 Proximal anteromedial portal
2 Posterolateral portal
3 Posterocentral portal
4 Proximal anterolateral portal
5 Direct posterolateral portal (soft spot)

2.6.1 Proximal Anteromedial Portal

The proximal anteromedial portal is located anterior to the medial intermuscular septum and 2 cm proximal to the medial epicondyle. This portal allows an excellent view of the radiohumeral and most of the ulnohumeral joints. The advantage of this portal is its proximal location and the distal orientation of the arthroscope, almost parallel to the median nerve in the sagittal plane. However, one must be careful with the ulnar nerve as it is located posterior to the medial intermuscular septum, 3–4 mm away from the portal. The direct palpation of the septum and the anterior location of the portal decrease the risk of injury to this nerve (**Figs. 2.14–2.18**).

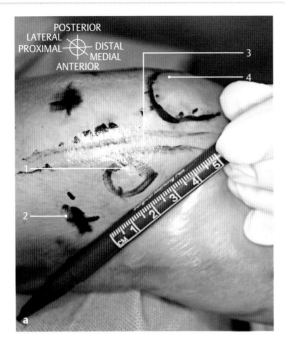

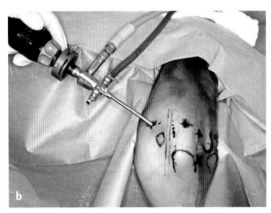

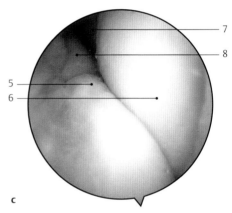

Fig. 2.14 Medial view of a right (cadaveric) elbow shows **(a)** the proximal anteromedial portal and **(b)** the position of the arthroscope. **(c)** Arthroscopic view.

1 Medial epicondyle
2 Proximal anteromedial portal
3 Ulnar nerve
4 Olecranon
5 Coronoid process
6 Trochlea of the humerus
7 Capitulum
8 Radial head

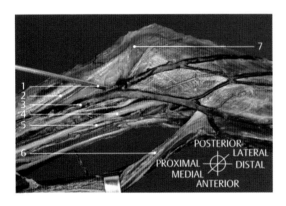

Fig. 2.15 Medial view of a right (cadaveric) elbow in a position similar to the lateral decubitus arthroscopic setting shows the proximal anteromedial portal marked with a Steinmann rod and the related anatomical structures.

1 Proximal anteromedial portal (Steinmann rod)
2 Medial intermuscular septum
3 Basilic vein
4 Median nerve
5 Brachial artery
6 Biceps muscle and tendon
7 Medial epicondyle

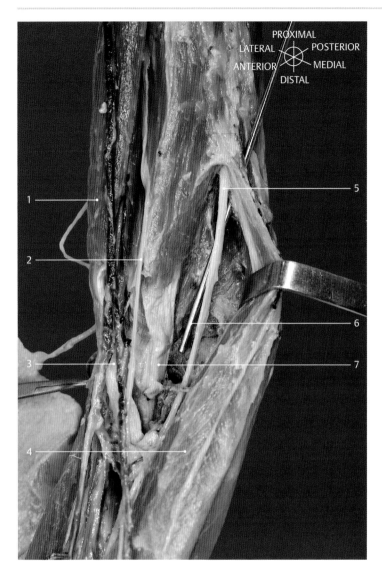

Fig. 2.16   Anterior view of a right (cadaveric) elbow shows the route of the arthroscope from the anteromedial portal to the elbow joint and the related anatomical structures.

1 Biceps muscle
2 Musculocutaneous nerve
3 Biceps muscle tendon
4 Pronator teres muscle
5 Median nerve
6 Steinmann rod in the proximal anteromedial portal
7 Brachialis muscle tendon

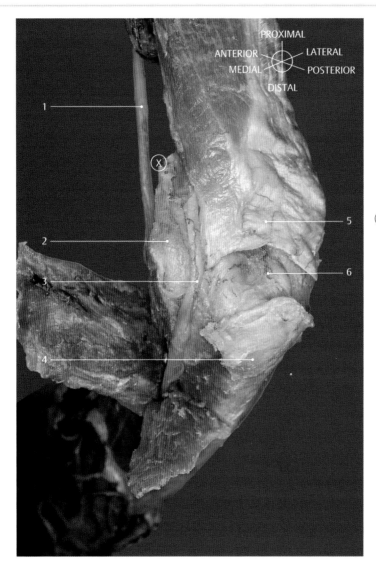

Fig. 2.17 Posterior view of a right (cadaveric) elbow shows the position of both the median and ulnar nerves to the proximal anteromedial portal.

1 Median nerve
2 Medial epicondyle
3 Ulnar nerve
4 Olecranon
5 Triceps brachii muscle tendon
6 Posterior joint capsule
Ⓧ Proximal anteromedial portal

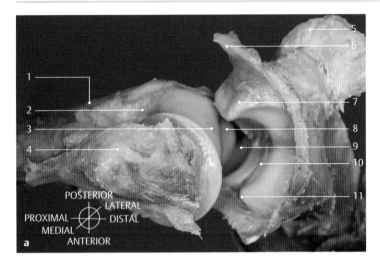

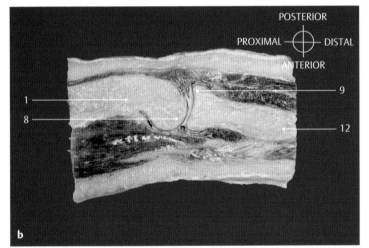

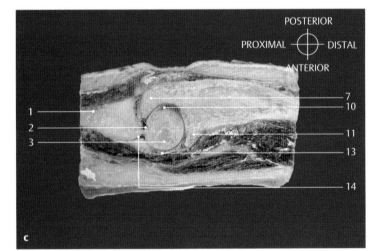

Fig. 2.18   (a–c) Osteoarticular structures and sagittal cuts of a right (cadaveric) elbow show the radiohumeral and ulnohumeral joints.

1 Distal humerus
2 Olecranon fossa
3 Trochlea of the humerus
4 Medial epicondyle
5 Triceps muscle tendon
6 Posterior capsule
7 Olecranon
8 Capitulum
9 Radial head
10 Trochlear notch
11 Coronoid process
12 Proximal radius
13 Anterior capsule
14 Coronoid fossa

2.6.2 Proximal Anterolateral Portal

The proximal anterolateral portal is located 1–2 cm proximal to the lateral epicondyle, directly over the anterior humerus, and allows access to the medial zone of the ulnohumeral joint, the radiohumeral joint, and the lateral recess. The radial nerve is the structure that is most frequently damaged during arthroscopic instrumentation of the elbow joint. However, the proximal location and its path along the longitudinal axis of the anterior part of the humerus reduces this risk (**Figs. 2.19–2.21**).

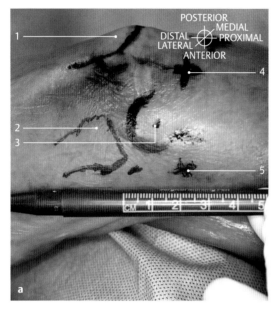

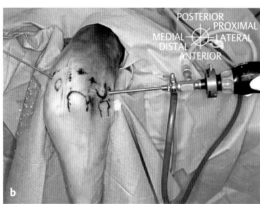

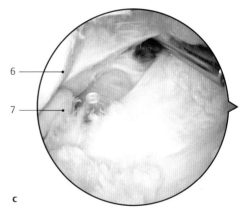

Fig. 2.19   Lateral and superolateral views of a right (cadaveric) elbow show the **(a)** anatomical osseous landmarks and **(b)** the position of the proximal anterolateral portal. **(c)** Shows the arthroscopic view.

1 Olecranon
2 Radial head
3 Capitulum/lateral epicondyle
4 Posterolateral portal
5 Proximal anterolateral portal
6 Trochlea of the humerus
7 Coronoid process

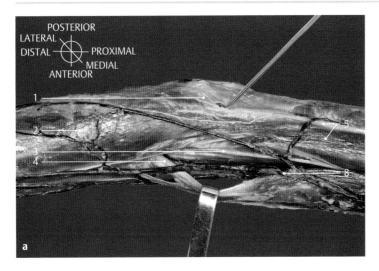

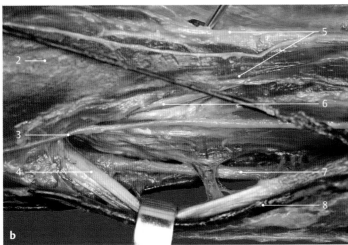

Fig. 2.20   A right (cadaveric) elbow in the lateral decubitus position; **(a)** the location of the proximal anterolateral portal is marked by a Steinmann rod and **(b)** the anterior anatomical structures at risk during arthroscopic instrumentation of the elbow are shown.

1 Lateral epicondyle
2 Brachioradialis muscle
3 Musculocutaneous/lateral cutaneous nerve of the forearm
4 Biceps muscle tendon
5 Brachialis muscle and lateral muscular septum
6 Radial nerve
7 Median nerve
8 Cephalic vein

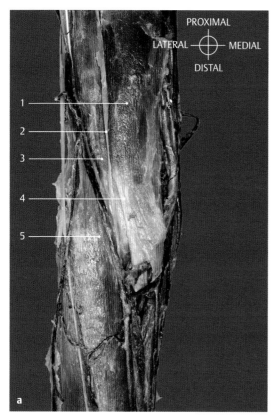

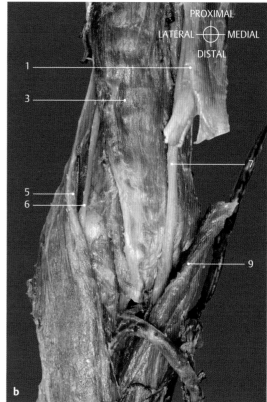

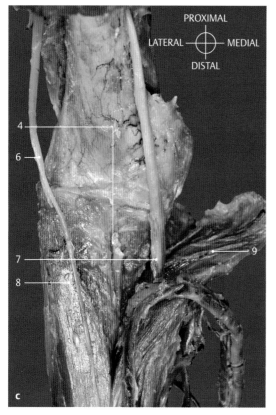

Fig. 2.21 **(a–c)** A sequence of images of a right (cadaveric) elbow shows the anterior nervous structures potentially at risk when using the proximal anterolateral portal.

1 Biceps muscle
2 Musculocutaneous/lateral antebrachial cutaneous nerve
3 Brachialis muscle
4 Biceps muscle tendon
5 Brachioradialis muscle
6 Radial nerve
7 Median nerve
8 Supinator muscle
9 Pronator teres muscle

2.6.3 Posterocentral Portal

The posterocentral portal is located 3 cm proximal to the tip of the olecranon at the midline of the elbow and allows an excellent view of the posterior compartment, the olecranon fossa, and the lateral and medial gutter. The posterior antebrachial cutaneous nerve and the ulnar nerve are located equidistant 25 mm to the posterocentral portal (**Figs. 2.22–2.24**).

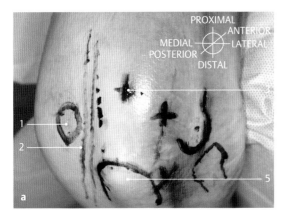

Fig. 2.22 Superior and posterior views of a right (cadaveric) elbow show the **(a)** anatomical landmarks and the **(b)** location of the posterocentral portal. **(c)** Shows the arthroscopic view.

1 Medial epicondyle
2 Ulnar nerve
3 Posterocentral portal
4 Trochlea of the humerus
5 Tip of the olecranon

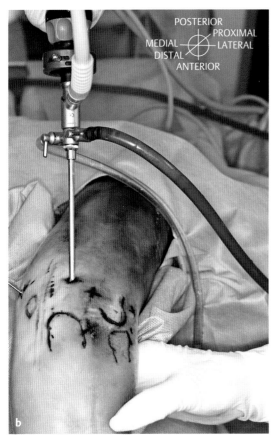

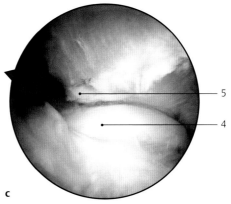

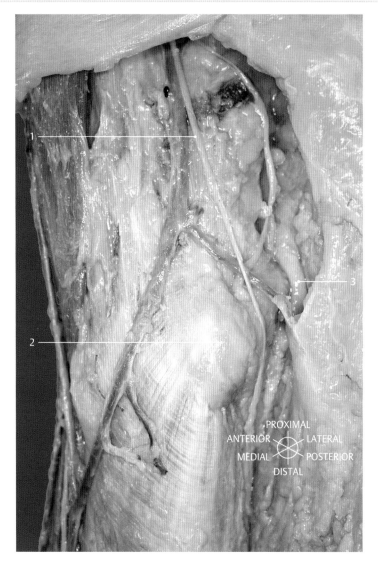

Fig. 2.23 Posteromedial view of a right (cadaveric) elbow shows the nerves at risk when using the posterocentral portal.

1 Medial antebrachial cutaneous nerve
2 Medial epicondyle
3 Ulnar nerve

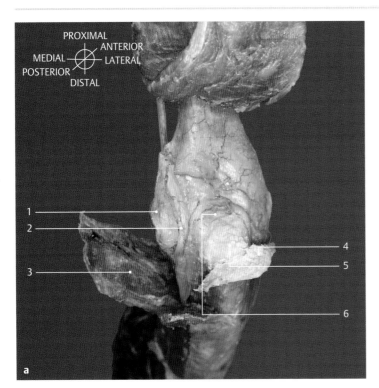

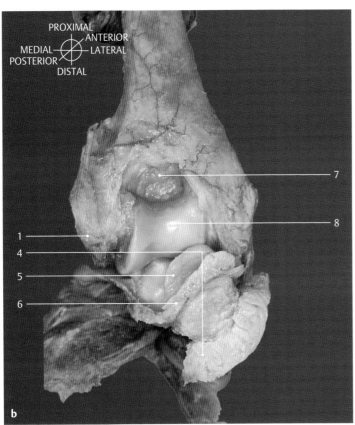

Fig. 2.24   (a, b) Images of a right (cadaveric) elbow (posterosuperior view) in which the relation of the osteoarticular structures with the ulnar nerve is evident.

1   Medial epicondyle
2   Ulnar nerve
3   Flexor carpi ulnaris
4   Triceps muscle tendon
5   Olecranon
6   Posterior joint capsule
7   Olecranon fossa
8   Trochlea of the humerus

2.6.4 Posterolateral Portal

The posterolateral portal of the elbow is located 2 cm proximal to the tip of the olecranon at the lateral border of the triceps muscle tendon and is used as an instrumentation portal during a posterior arthroscopy of the elbow. Through this portal it is possible to get access to the tip of the olecranon, the olecranon fossa, and the posterior trochlea. However, it is not possible to get access to the posterior capitulum (**Fig. 2.25**).

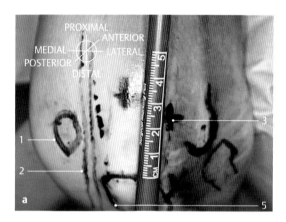

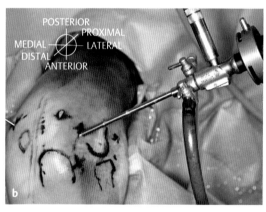

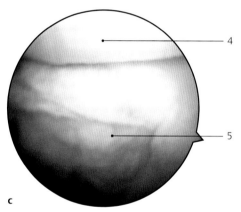

Fig. 2.25 **(a)** Posterosuperior view a right (cadaveric) elbow with the anatomical landmarks marked and **(b)** the arthroscope in the posterolateral portal. **(c)** Shows the arthroscopic view.

1 Medial epicondyle
2 Ulnar nerve
3 Posterolateral portal
4 Trochlea of the humerus
5 Olecranon

2.6.5 Direct Posterolateral Portal or Soft Spot

The direct posterolateral portal is located in the center of a triangle formed by the lateral epicondyle, the olecranon, and the radial head. This location is used to distend the joint with saline solution before performing the first portal. When used as a visualization portal, it allows access to the inferior capitulum and the proximal radioulnar joint. The inferior lateral cutaneous nerve of the arm (radial nerve branch) is at risk when using this portal, as it is located 7 mm from the portal site (**Figs. 2.26–2.29**).

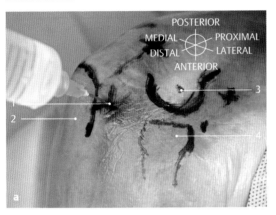

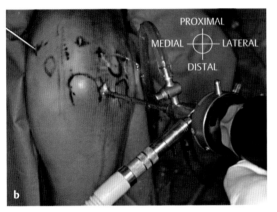

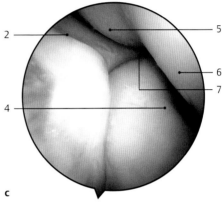

Fig. 2.26 **(a)** Posterolateral view of a right (cadaveric) elbow shows the anatomical landmarks and the **(b)** arthroscope in the direct posterolateral portal. **(c)** Shows the arthroscopic view.

1 Hypodermic needle in the direct posterolateral portal
2 Trochlear notch
3 Lateral epicondyle
4 Radial head
5 Trochlea of the humerus
6 Capitulum
7 Proximal radioulnar joint

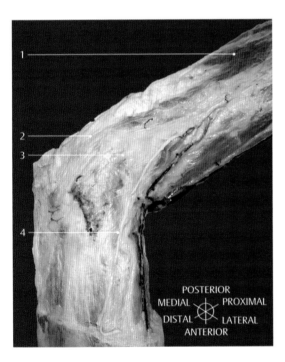

Fig. 2.27   Lateral view of a right (cadaveric) elbow in a similar setting to the lateral decubitus position shows the location of the posterior cutaneous nerve of the forearm (radial nerve branch).

1 Triceps brachii muscle
2 Olecranon
3 Lateral epicondyle
4 Inferior lateral cutaneous nerve of the arm

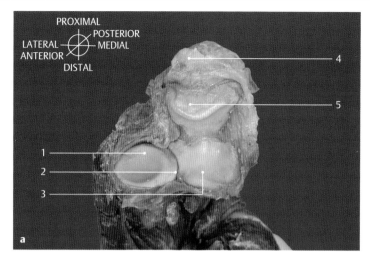

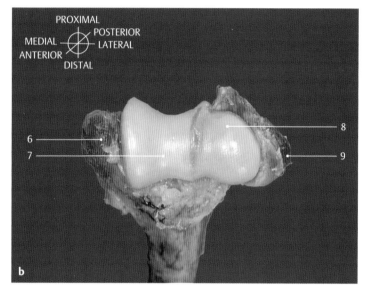

Fig. 2.28   (a, b) Articular structures of the elbow that can be evaluated using the direct posterolateral portal: the inferior zone of the capitulum and the proximal radioulnar joint.

1 Radial head
2 Proximal radioulnar joint
3 Trochlear notch
4 Posterior joint capsule
5 Olecranon
6 Medial epicondyle
7 Trochlea of the humerus
8 Capitulum
9 Lateral epicondyle

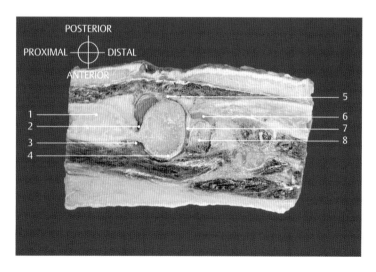

Fig. 2.29 Sagittal cut of a right (cadaveric) elbow.

1 Distal humerus
2 Olecranon fossa
3 Coronoid fossa
4 Trochlea of the humerus
5 Trochlear notch
6 Radial notch
7 Coronoid process
8 Radial head

2.7 Suggested Sequence for an Elbow Arthroscopy

To perform a complete arthroscopic evaluation of the elbow joint a thorough and methodical exam ination is advised. In general a 30-degree standard 4-mm arthroscope is recommended for adults and a 2.7-mm scope is used in teenagers and infants. The patient is put in the lateral decubitus position, the use of a tourniquet is recommended, and the external landmarks are established with a sterile draping in place. The ulnar nerve is checked to rule out instability by flexion and extension of the elbow.

The joint is distended with 20–30 mL of saline solution through the direct posterolateral portal zone, which moves the neurovascular structures away from the anterior capsule. Over-distention of the joint should be avoided to prevent the rupture of the capsule. The arthroscopic techniques for the anterior and posterior compartments and the posterolateral recess are described in the following text.

2.8 Arthroscopy of the Anterior Compartment of the Elbow

Pathologies treated arthroscopically in the anterior compartment of the elbow include synovitis; chondral lesions of the capitulum, trochlea, radial head, and coronoid process; the removal of loose bodies; and osteophytes, capsular releases, lateral epicondylopathy, and synovial folds.

Once the arthroscope is installed in the proximal anteromedial portal, the first step is the evaluation of the radiohumeral joint. This is identified by pronosupination of the radial head (**Fig. 2.30**).

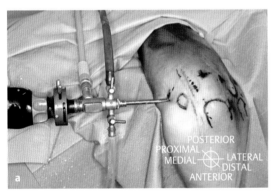

Fig. 2.30 **(a)** View of a right (cadaveric) elbow. The arthroscope is in the proximal anteromedial portal, with the lens rotated to look at the most lateral portion of the anterior compartment. **(b, c)** Show the arthroscopic views.

1 Anterior capitulum
2 Radial head
3 Synovial capsule, anterolateral and distal portion

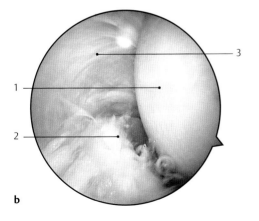

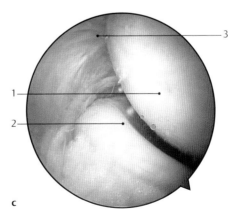

From the position shown in **Fig. 2.30**, the lens of the arthroscope should be rotated for the evaluation of the lateral aspect of the joint capsule and its insertion from proximal to distal (**Fig. 2.31**).

Next, slowly take out the arthroscope and keep the lens looking distal, thus allowing for the evaluation of the ulnohumeral joint (**Fig. 2.32**).

From the previous position, the lens is rotated to evaluate the coronoid fossa (**Fig. 2.33**).

The evaluation of the most medial part of the joint capsule and its proximal and distal attachment in the coronoid process is done by simple rotations of the lens (**Fig. 2.34**).

Next, the proximal anterolateral portal is established via direct arthroscopic control from the proximal anteromedial portal. This portal can be used for instrumentation or visualization purposes (**Fig. 2.35**).

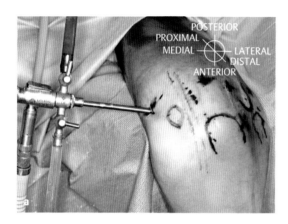 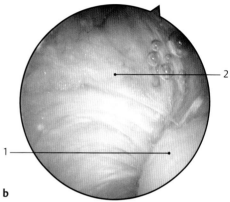

Fig. 2.31　(**a**) A right (cadaveric) elbow with the arthroscope in the proximal anteromedial portal for an evaluation of the lateral and proximal portion of the anterior capsule. (**b**) Arthroscopic view.

1 Capitulum, 2 Joint capsule

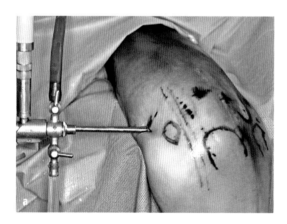 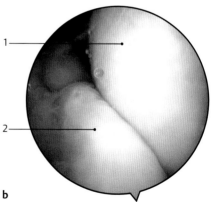

Fig. 2.32　(**a**) A right (cadaveric) elbow with the location of the arthroscope and lens in the proximal anteromedial portal for an evaluation of the coronoid process and humeral trochlea. (**b**) Arthroscopic view.

1 Humeral trochlea, 2 Coronoid process

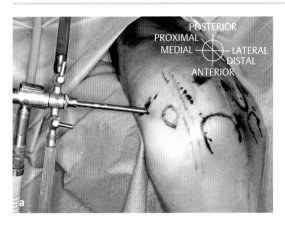
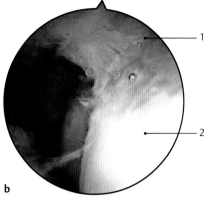

Fig. 2.33 **(a)** A right (cadaveric) elbow with the arthroscope in the proximal anteromedial portal and the rotation of the lens to evaluate the coronoid fossa and humeral trochlea. **(b)** Arthroscopic view.

1 Coronoid fossa, 2 Humeral trochlea

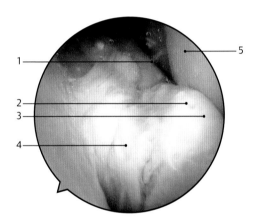

Fig. 2.34 Arthroscopic view of a right elbow from the proximal anteromedial portal shows the insertion of the distal and proximal capsule to the coronoid process.

1 Radial head
2 Coronoid process
3 Proximal joint capsule
4 Distal joint capsule
5 Trochlea of the humerus

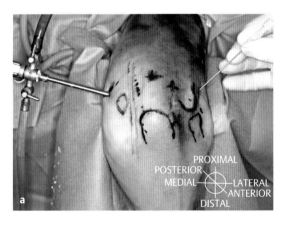
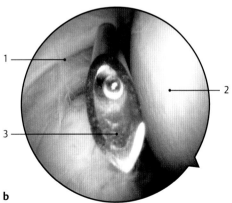

Fig. 2.35 **(a)** A right (cadaveric) elbow shows the correct location of the proximal anterolateral portal under arthroscopic control from the proximal anteromedial portal and the lens looking toward the capitulum and proximal lateral joint capsule. **(b)** Arthroscopic view.

1 Proximal lateral capsule, 2 Capitulum, 3 Spinal needle

Once this sequence is complete, the arthroscope can be switched to the proximal anterolateral portal. We suggest using a Steinmann rod (**Fig. 2.36**).

Through the proximal anterolateral portal it is possible to get a better evaluation of the most medial portion of the ulnohumeral joint, and to use the proximal anteromedial portal for instrumentation purposes (**Fig. 2.37**).

Once this sequence is complete, you can proceed with the specific procedure.

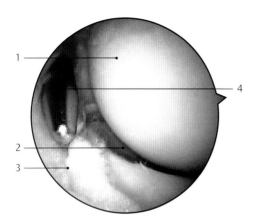

Fig. 2.36   Arthroscopic view of a right elbow from the proximal anteromedial portal. A 'Steinmann' rod is used to guide the arthroscopic cannula through the proximal anterolateral portal.

1 Capitulum
2 Radial head
3 Joint capsule
4 Steinmann rod

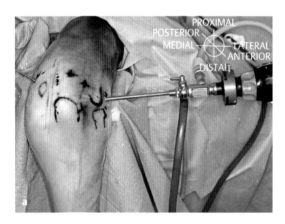

Fig. 2.37   (a) A right (cadaveric) elbow with the arthroscopic view from the proximal anterolateral portal shows the right location of the arthroscope and lens rotation for a proper evaluation of the most medial part of the anterior compartment of the elbow. A Steinmann rod is left in the proximal anteromedial portal in case it is needed again. **(b, c)** Arthroscopic views.

1 Capitulum, 2 Radial head, 3 Trochlea of the humerus, 4 Coronoid process, 5 Steinmann rod in the proximal anteromedial portal, 6 Medial joint capsule

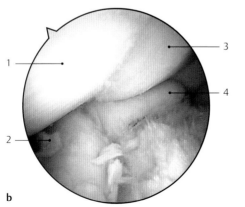

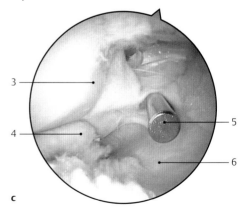

2.9   Arthroscopy of the Posterior Compartment of the Elbow

The pathologies treated via posterior arthroscopy of the elbow include synovitis, synovial pathology, osteochondral lesions of the capitulum, osteophytes and loose body removal, capsular releases, and posteromedial or posterolateral impingements.

The posterocentral portal is established first; the arthroscope is inserted toward the olecranon fossa and the correct location is confirmed by feeling an osseous stop. It is suggested to leave a Steinmann rod or trocar in the proximal anteromedial portal in case it is needed again and to avoid over-distention of the joint during long surgeries (**Fig. 2.38**).

Next, identify the olecranon and obtain a view of the olecranon fossa by flexion and extension of the elbow (**Fig. 2.39**).

From this starting position, the lens is rotated to evaluate the posterolateral and medial gutters. This is easier after a slight elbow extension (**Fig. 2.40**).

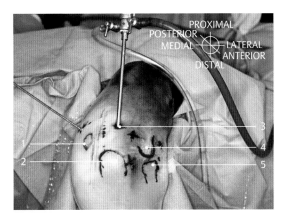

Fig. 2.38   A right (cadaveric) elbow, with the arthroscope in the posterocentral portal pointing toward the olecranon fossa.

1   Medial epicondyle
2   Olecranon
3   Posterocentral portal
4   Lateral epicondyle
5   Radial head

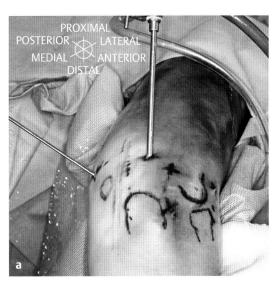

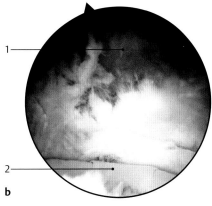

Fig. 2.39   **(a)** A right (cadaveric) elbow with the arthroscope in the posterocentral portal and the lens in the correct rotation for an evaluation of the tip of the olecranon and the olecranon fossa. **(b)** Arthroscopic view.

1 Olecranon fossa, 2 Tip of the olecranon

57

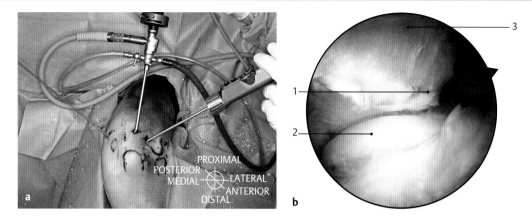

Fig. 2.40 **(a)** A right (cadaveric) elbow with the arthroscope in the posterocentral portal and the lens rotated to get a view of the posterior gutters. **(b)** Arthroscopic view.

1 Olecranon, 2 Trochlea of the humerus, 3 Posterior joint capsule

2.10 Arthroscopy of the Lateral Recess of the Elbow

The direct posterolateral portal (soft spot) can be established under direct arthroscopic control from the posterocentral or posterolateral portal using a spinal needle (**Fig. 2.41**).

Through the direct posterolateral portal it is possible to evaluate the posterior ulnohumeral articular cartilage, the inferior portion of the capitulum, and the proximal radioulnar joint (**Fig. 2.42**).

Once this sequence is complete, you can proceed with the planned procedure.

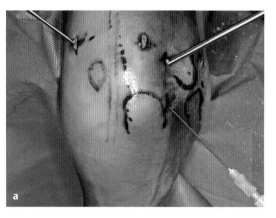
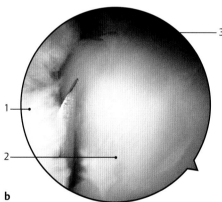

Fig. 2.41 **(a)** A right elbow with the arthroscope in the posterolateral portal and the lens looking toward the posterolateral border of the olecranon to confirm the correct entry of the spinal needle (distal to proximal) through the direct posterolateral portal (soft spot). **(b)** Arthroscopic view.

1 Olecranon (posterolateral), 2 Trochlea, 3 Olecranon fossa

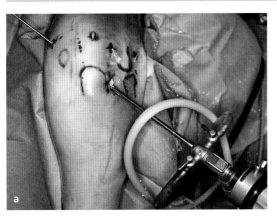

Fig. 2.42 **(a)** A right (cadaveric) elbow with the arthroscope in the direct posterolateral portal to evaluate the posterior ulnohumeral joint, the proximal radioulnar joint, and the inferior portion of the capitulum. **(b, c)** Arthroscopic views.

1 Trochlea of the humerus
2 Trochlear notch of the proximal ulna
3 Capitulum
4 Radial notch of the proximal ulna
5 Radial head

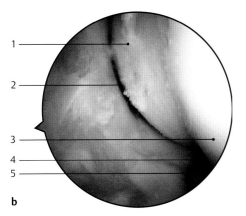

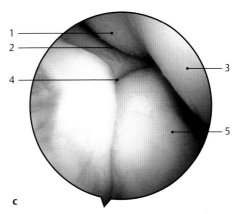

3 Wrist

Cristian Blanco Moreno, Gonzalo Espinoza Lavín, Juan Eduardo Santorcuato Fuentes, Eduardo Leopold González, and Carlos Espech López

3.1 Introduction

Wrist arthroscopy is a technique that allows a view of the inner anatomy of the wrist (the radiocarpal and midcarpal joints) with minimum surgical damage to the tissues, which allows for more precise diagnostic powers and less aggressive treatment of wrist joint pathologies as compared to traditional open techniques. Wrist arthroscopy is complex and complications are possible; however, many of these complications can be prevented with an accurate knowledge of this joint's anatomy. This chapter presents the different dorsal portals for the radiocarpal and midcarpal joints and the related anatomy.

3.2 Patient Positioning

Wrist arthroscopy is performed under regional or general anesthesia. The use of a tourniquet is optional, depending on the pathology to be treated. The patient is placed supine on the table with the elbow flexed to 90 degrees and the hand suspended from the traction tower with sterile finger traps on the index and/or middle finger. Apply traction weight, usually 2–3 kg, for a gentle distraction of the joint **(Fig. 3.1).**

3.3 Basic Technique for an Arthroscopic Examination of the Wrist

3.3.1 Radiocarpal Joint

The arthroscopic evaluation of the radiocarpal joint starts with portal 3–4. Then portal 4–5 is established under direct arthroscopic control. Portal 4–5 is used primarily for the palpatory evaluation of the radiocarpal joint. After this is complete, you can switch portals for an additional view and palpation of the radiocarpal joint. Portals 6R and 6U are used for the evaluation, instrumentation, and repair procedures of the articular disk (triangular fibrocartilage). Portal 1–2 is used less frequently, but is helpful to evaluate the most radial and distal zone of the scaphoid.

3.3.2 Midcarpal Joint

The arthroscopic evaluation of the midcarpal joint starts at the radial midcarpal portal (distal to the radiocarpal portal 3–4), then under direct arthroscopic control the ulnar midcarpal portal (distal to the radiocarpal portal 4–5) is established. After this is complete, you can switch portals for an additional view and palpation of the midcarpal joint, as with the radiocarpal joint. The arthroscopic evaluation of the midcarpal joint is routinely done for intercarpal instability cases.

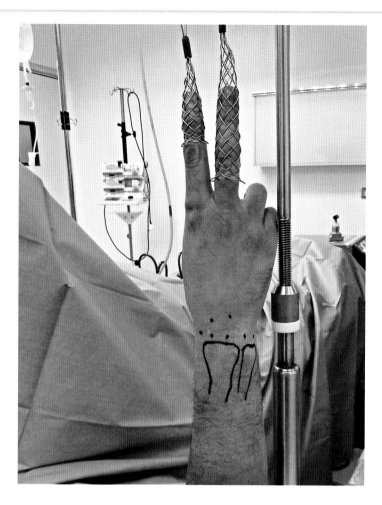

Fig. 3.1 The traction tower stabilizes the forearm and allows distraction of the wrist joint.

3.3.3 Dorsal Anatomy of the Wrist

A detailed knowledge of the anatomy of the wrist is key for an adequate portal placement. Neurovascular and tendinous structures are at risk during wrist arthroscopy. The superficial landmarks and the tendinous and osteoarticular structures of the wrist are shown in **Figs. 3.2–3.6.**

3.4 General Indications for a Wrist Arthroscopy

The therapeutic indications for a wrist arthroscopy include:

- Diagnostic arthroscopy for chronic pain
- Articular disk (triangular fibrocartilage) lesions (reinsertions in peripheral lesions, central debridements, sutures)
- Scapholunate ligament lesions
- Chondral lesions
- Synovitis
- Ganglions
- Loose bodies
- Arthroscopic assistance in reduction and fixation of distal radius and scaphoid fractures

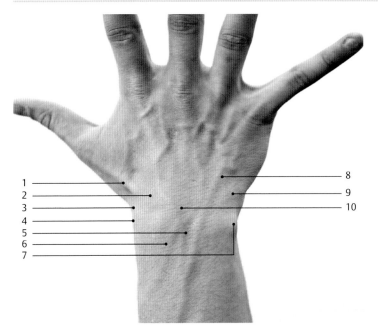

Fig. 3.2 Dorsal view of a right wrist.

1 Extensor pollicis longus
2 Extensor carpi radialis longus and brevis
3 Extensor pollicis brevis and abductor pollicis longus
4 Radial artery
5 Dorsal tubercle of the radius (Lister's tubercle)
6 Distal radius
7 Distal ulna
8 Extensor digiti minimi
9 Extensor carpi ulnaris
10 Extensor digitorum and extensor indicis

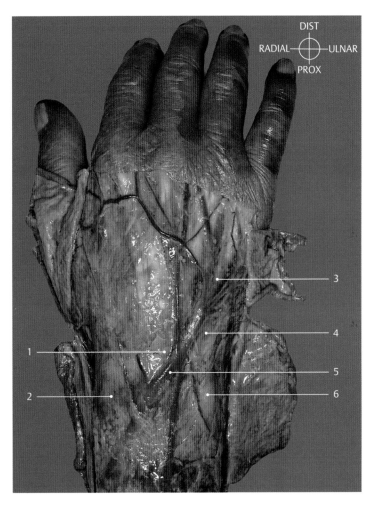

Fig. 3.3 Right wrist dissection shows the dorsal venous network.

1 Extensor digitorum
2 Distal radius
3 Extensor digiti minimi
4 Extensor carpi ulnaris
5 Cephalic vein
6 Distal ulna

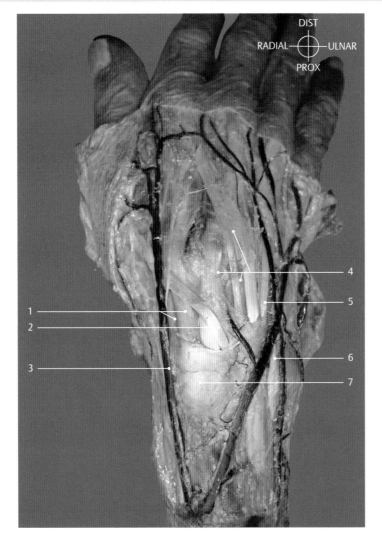

Fig. 3.4 Right wrist shows the dorsal tendinous layer.

1 Extensor carpi radiales brevis and longus
2 Extensor pollicis longus
3 Cephalic vein
4 Extensor digiti and extensor indicis
5 Extensor digiti minimi
6 Extensor carpi ulnaris
7 Extensor retinaculum

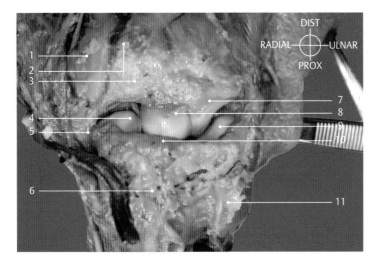

Fig. 3.5 Right wrist with the dorsal capsule opened to expose the distal row of the carpus and midcarpal joint.

1 Second metacarpal bone
2 Third metacarpal bone
3 Trapezoid
4 Scaphoid
5 Scaphotrapezium-trapezoid ligament
6 Distal radius
7 Hamate
8 Capitate
9 Triquetrum
10 Dorsal intercarpal ligament
11 Distal ulna

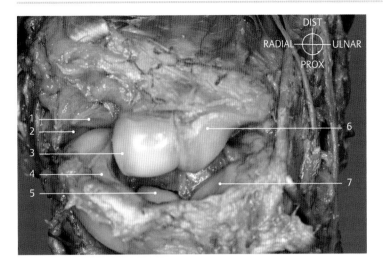

Fig. 3.6 Dorsal view of right wrist with the capsule opened at the midcarpal and radiocarpal joints to show the proximal and distal carpal rows.

1 Trapezoid
2 Trapezium
3 Capitate
4 Scaphoid
5 Lunate
6 Hamate
7 Triquetrum

3.5 Dorsal Arthroscopic Portals of the Wrist

The dorsal portals of the wrist are related to the dorsal extensor tendons compartments. The following description is based on this anatomical fact (**Figs. 3.7–3.11**). Each of the dorsal portals is analyzed according to the external anatomical landmarks, the anatomical structures at risk for the specific portal, and the intra-articular anatomy.

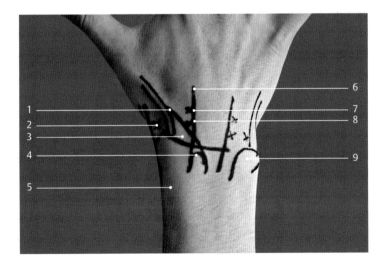

Fig. 3.7 Right wrist with the dorsal radial arthroscopic portals and main anatomical landmarks marked.

1 Extensor pollicis longus
2 Portal 1–2
3 Extensor carpi radiales brevis and longus
4 Dorsal tubercle of the radius (Lister's tubercle)
5 Distal radius
6 Extensor digitorum and extensor indicis
7 Radial midcarpal portal
8 Portal 3–4
9 Distal ulna

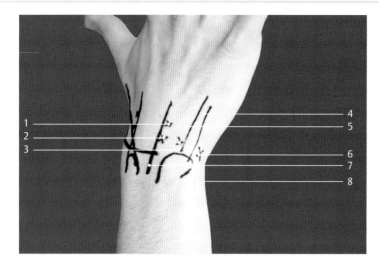

Fig. 3.8 Dorsoulnar view of right wrist with the ulnar portals and landmarks marked.

1 Ulnar midcarpal portal
2 Portal 4–5
3 Portal 6R
4 Extensor carpi ulnaris
5 Extensor digiti minimi
6 Portal 6U
7 Extensor digitorum
8 Distal ulna

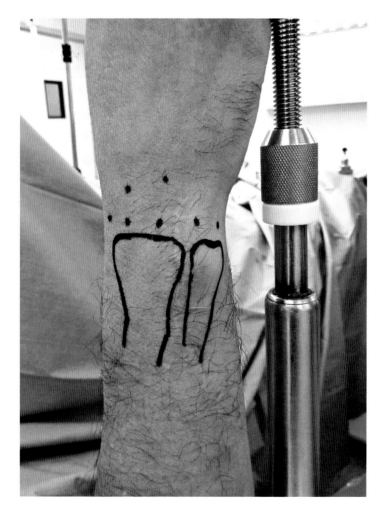

Fig. 3.9 Right wrist positioned for a surgical procedure shows the location of the dorsal portals in this setting.

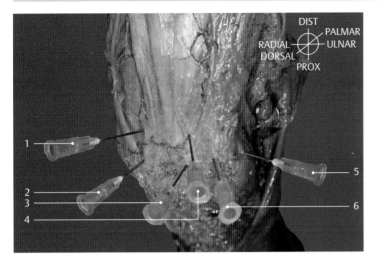

Fig. 3.10 Dorsal view of right wrist showing the position of the dorsal portals (except portal 1–2).

1 Radial midcarpal portal
2 Portal 3–4
3 Portal 4–5
4 Ulnar midcarpal portal
5 Portal 6U
6 Portal 6R

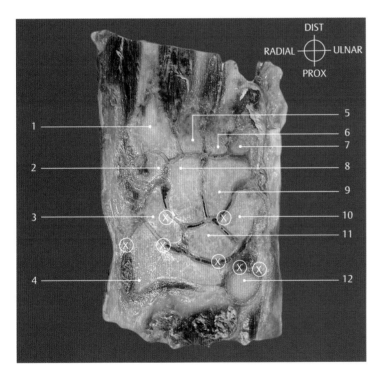

Fig. 3.11 Frontal cut of right wrist showing the osseous and articular anatomy of the carpus.

1 Second metacarpal bone
2 Trapezoid
3 Scaphoid
4 Distal radius
5 Third metacarpal bone
6 Fourth metacarpal bone
7 Fifth metacarpal bone
8 Capitate
9 Hamate
10 Triquetrum
11 Lunate
12 Distal ulna
ⓧ Portals

3.5.1 Portal 1–2

Portal 1–2 is located between the extensor compartments 1 (abductor pollicis longus and extensor pollicis brevis) and 2 (extensor carpi radiales brevis and longus). The external anatomical landmarks are shown in **Figs. 3.12** and **3.13.**

Anatomy and Structures at Risk

The anatomical structures at risk when establishing portal 1–2 are the same tendons that define its location: the sensitive branch of the radial nerve and the radial artery. **Figs. 3.14–3.17** show the relevant anatomy for this portal. **Figs. 3.18** and **3.19** show different views of the radiocarpal joint using portal 1-2.

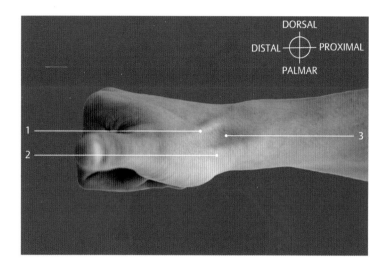

Fig. 3.12   Radial view of right wrist that shows the extensor compartments 1 and 2 (as well as the extensor pollicis longus).

1 Extensor pollicis longus
2 Abductor pollicis longus and extensor pollicis brevis
3 Extensor carpi radiales brevis and longus

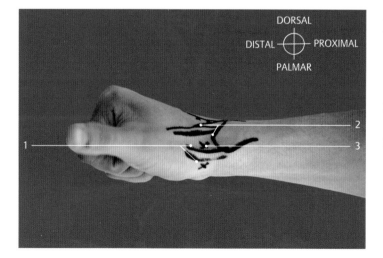

Fig. 3.13   Right wrist shows the superficial landmarks for the portal 1–2.

1 Abductor pollicis longus and extensor pollicis brevis
2 Extensor carpi radiales brevis and longus
3 Portal 1–2

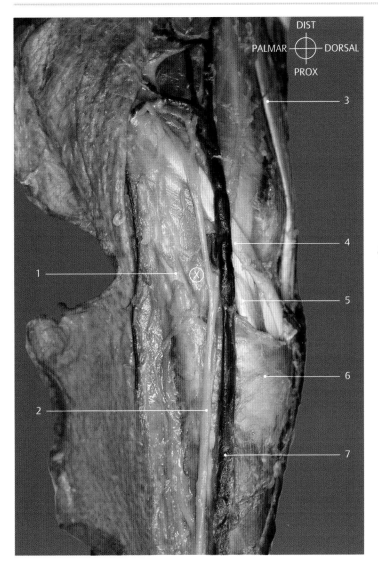

Fig. 3.14   Radial view of right wrist shows the relevant structures for the portal 1–2.

1 Abductor pollicis longus and extensor pollicis brevis
2 Superficial branch of the radial nerve
3 Extensor digitorum/indicis
4 Extensor pollicis longus
5 Extensor carpi radiales brevis and longus
6 Extensor retinaculum
7 Cephalic vein
(X) Portal 1–2

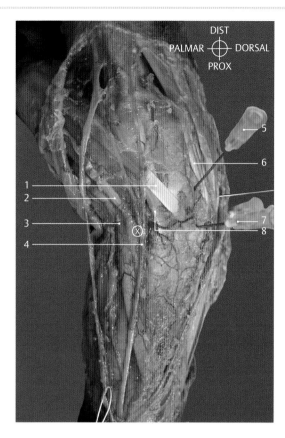

Fig. 3.15 Radial view of right wrist shows the area for portal 1–2 and its topographic relation with other portals (portal 3–4 and the radial midcarpal portal).

1 Extensor pollicis longus
2 Extensor pollicis brevis
3 Abductor pollicis longus
4 Superficial branch of the radial nerve
5 Radial midcarpal portal
6 Extensor digitorum
7 Portal 3–4
8 Extensor carpi radiales brevis and longus
ⓧ Portal 1–2

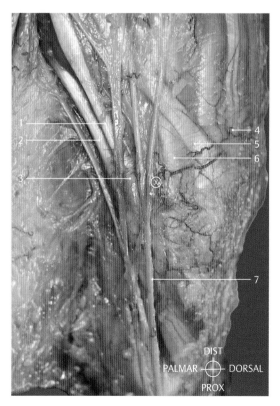

Fig. 3.16 Radial view of right wrist shows the radial anatomy and the position of portal 1–2.

1 Extensor pollicis brevis
2 Abductor pollicis longus
3 Radial artery
4 Extensor digitorum
5 Extensor pollicis longus
6 Extensor carpi radialis longus and brevis
7 Superficial branches of the radial nerve
ⓧ Portal 1–2

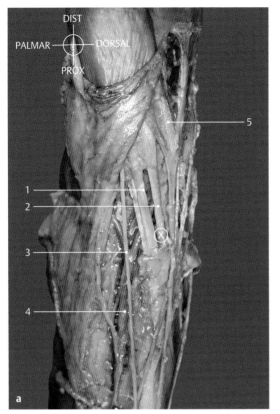

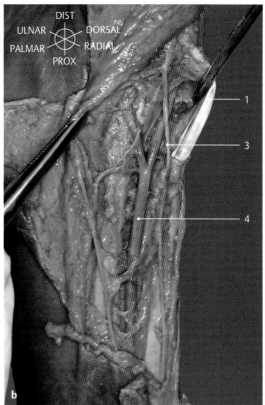

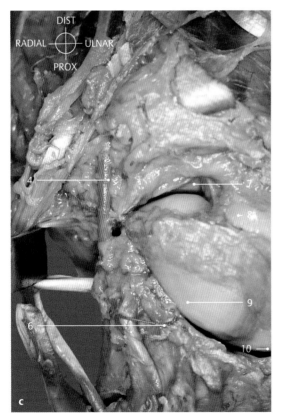

Fig. 3.17 (a–c) Anatomy of the radial artery as related to portal 1–2: radial view, palmar view, and finally part of the radial artery at the level of the first and second carpal row.

1 Abductor pollicis longus and extensor pollicis brevis
2 Extensor carpi radiales brevis and longus
3 Superficial branch of the radial nerve
4 Radial artery
5 Extensor pollicis longus
6 Distal radius
7 Trapezoid
8 Capitate
9 Scaphoid
10 Lunate
ⓧ Portal 1–2

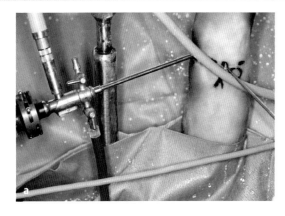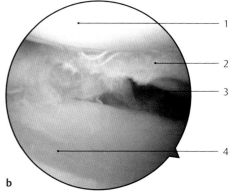

Fig. 3.18 **(a)** Right wrist with the arthroscope in portal 1–2 as the lens looks ulnar. **(b)** Arthroscopic view.

1 Scaphoid, 2 Scapholunate ligament, 3 Lunate, 4 Distal radius

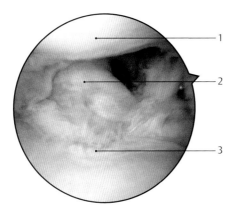

Fig. 3.19 Arthroscopic view of right wrist with the arthroscope in portal 1–2 as the lens looks dorsal and ulnar.

1 Lunate
2 Palmar long radiolunate ligament
3 Distal radius

3.5.2 Portal 3–4

Portal 3–4 is located between the extensor compartments 3 (extensor pollicis longus) and 4 (extensor digitorum–extensor indicis), distal to the dorsal tubercle of radius (Lister's tubercle). This is the main portal for wrist arthroscopy at the radiocarpal joint because it enters at the scapholunate interval. The external anatomical landmarks are shown in **Fig. 3.20**.

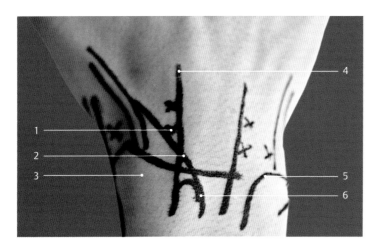

Fig. 3.20 Dorsal view of right wrist shows the external landmarks.

1 Portal 3–4
2 Extensor pollicis longus
3 Distal radius
4 Extensor digitorum
5 Distal ulna
6 Dorsal tubercle of radius (Lister's tubercle)

Anatomy and Structures at Risk

The structures at risk are the same tendons that define the location of portal 3–4. **Figs. 3.21–3.23** show the related anatomy for portal 3–4.

The radiocarpal joint is examined via portal 3–4. **Figs. 3.24** and **3.25** show the articular anatomy of the radiocarpal joint using this portal.

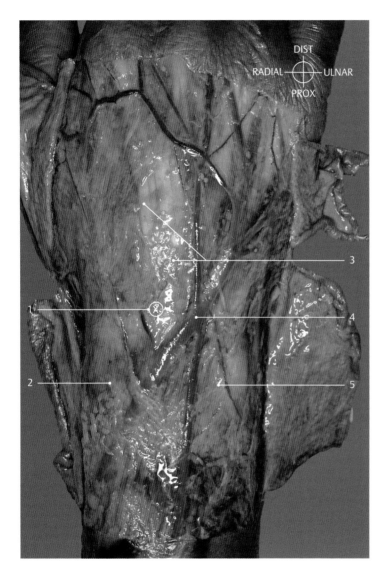

Fig. 3.21   Dorsal view of right wrist shows the subcutaneous structures.

1 (x) Portal 3–4
2 Distal radius
3 Extensor digitorum/extensor indicis
4 Dorsal venous network
5 Distal ulna

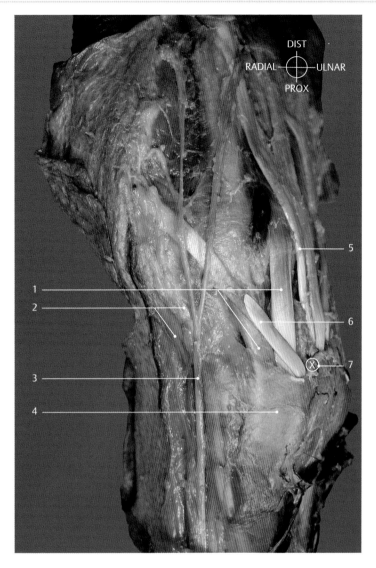

Fig. 3.22 Dorsal view of right wrist shows the tendinous structures for portal 3–4.

1 Extensor carpi radiales brevis and longus
2 Abductor pollicis longus and extensor pollicis brevis
3 Superficial branch of the radial nerve
4 Extensor retinaculum
5 Extensor digitorum/extensor indicis
6 Extensor pollicis longus
7 (X) Portal 3–4

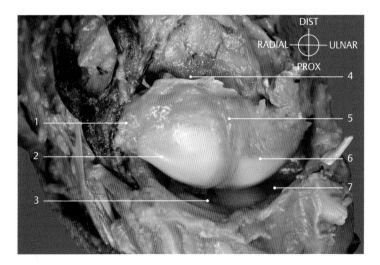

Fig. 3.23 Dorsoradial view of right wrist shows the open radiocarpal joint and the articular structures to be examined via the portal 3–4.

1 Scaphotrapezio-trapezoid ligament
2 Scaphoid
3 Distal radius
4 Midcarpal joint
5 Scapholunate ligament,
6 Lunate
7 Distal ulna

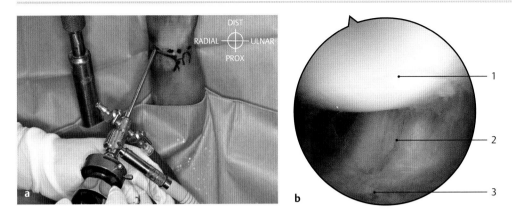

Fig. 3.24   (a) Right wrist with the arthroscope in portal 3–4 as the lens looks radial. **(b)** Arthroscopic view.

1 Scaphoid, 2 Palmar long radiolunate ligament, 3 Distal radius

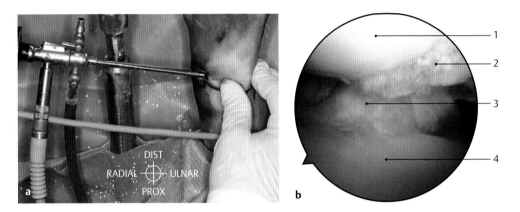

Fig. 3.25   (a) Right wrist with the arthroscope portal 3–4 as the lens looks palmar. **(b)** Arthroscopic view.

1 Scaphoid, 2 Scapholunate ligament, 3 Palmar long radiolunate ligament, 4 Distal radius

3.5.3 Portal 4–5

Portal 4–5 is located between the extensor compartment 4 (extensor digitorum, extensor indicis) and 5 (extensor digiti minimi) and is in line with the axis of the fourth metacarpal bone. This portal enters at the level of the midportion of the triangular fibrocartilage, and is the primary accessory portal for the instrumentation and evaluation of the radial portion of the radiocarpal joint. The external anatomical landmarks are shown in **Fig. 3.26**.

Anatomy and Structures at Risk

The structures at risk are the same tendons that define the location of portal 4–5. **Figs. 3.27–3.29** show the relevant anatomy for this portal. **Figs. 3.30–3.36** show different views of the radiocarpal joint using portal 4–5.

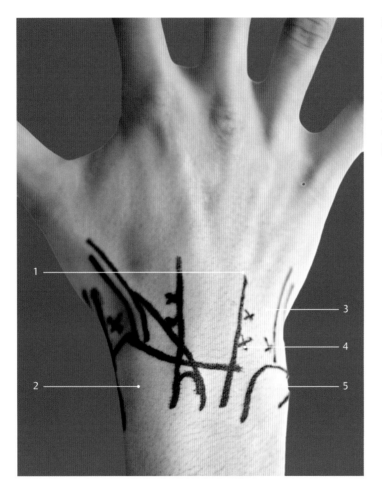

Fig. 3.26 Dorsal view of right wrist showing the external landmarks.

1 Extensor digitorum
2 Distal radius
3 Extensor digiti minimi
4 Portal 4–5
5 Distal ulna

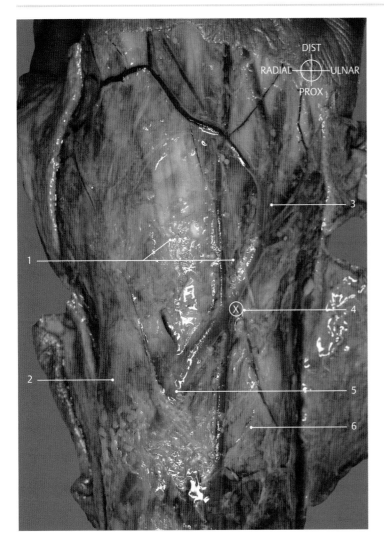

Fig. 3.27 Dorsal view of right wrist shows the subcutaneous structures and location for portal 4–5.

1 Extensor digitorum
2 Distal radius
3 Extensor digiti minimi
4 (X) Portal 4–5
5 Dorsal venous network
6 Distal ulna

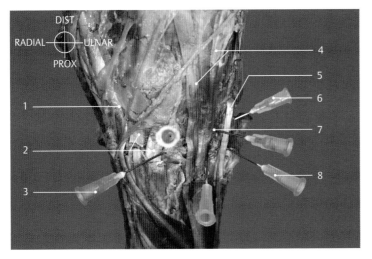

Fig. 3.28 Dorsal view of right wrist shows the dorsal tendons (extensor digitorum and extensor digiti minimi). The dorsal portals are marked with hypodermic needles, and note portal 4–5.

1 Extensor pollicis longus (displaced)
2 Extensor carpi radiales brevis and longus
3 Portal 3–4
4 Extensor digitorum
5 Extensor digiti minimi
6 Portal 6U
7 Portal 4–5
8 Portal 6R

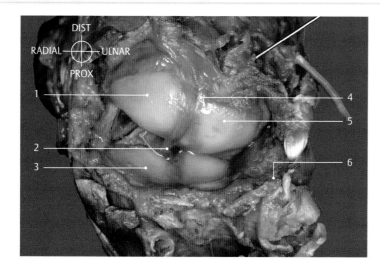

Fig. 3.29 Dorsal view of right wrist with the radiocarpal joint opened to show the articular structures to be examined via portal 4–5.

1 Scaphoid
2 Palmar long radiolunate ligament
3 Distal radius
4 Scapholunate ligament
5 Lunate
6 Distal ulna

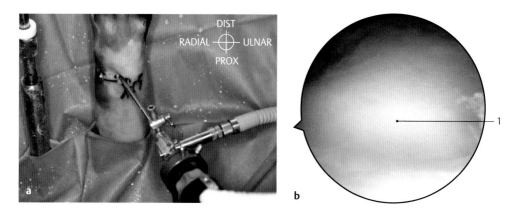

Fig. 3.30   (a) Right wrist with the arthroscope in portal 4–5 as the lens looks radial. **(b)** Arthroscopic view.
1 Distal radius

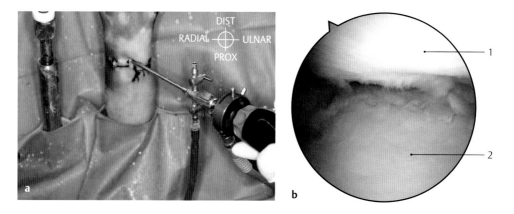

Fig. 3.31   (a) Right wrist with the arthroscope in portal 4–5 as the lens looks distal. **(b)** Arthroscopic view.
1 Scaphoid, 2 Distal radius

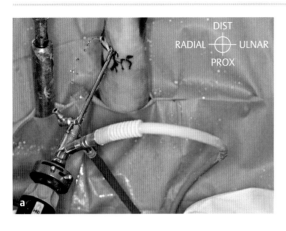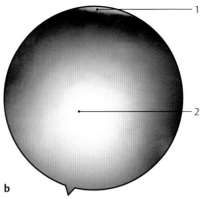

Fig. 3.32   (a) Right wrist with the arthroscope in portal 4–5 as the lens looks radial and proximal. **(b)** Arthroscopic view.

1 Scaphoid, 2 Distal radius

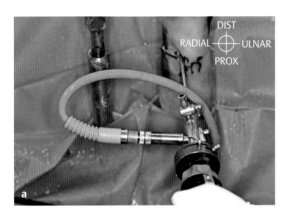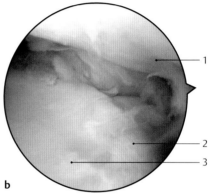

Fig. 3.33   (a) Right wrist with the arthroscope in portal 4–5 as the lens looks ulnar. **(b)** Arthroscopic view.

1 Lunate, 2 Articular disk (triangular fibrocartilage), 3 Distal radius

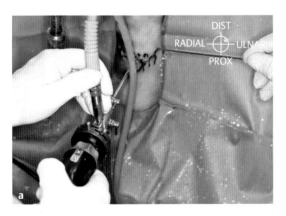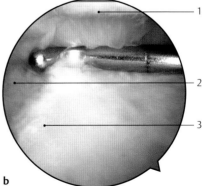

Fig. 3.34   (a) Right wrist with the arthroscope in portal 4–5 as the lens looks proximal and ulnar. **(b)** Arthroscopic view.

1 Lunate, 2 Distal radius, 3 Articular disk (triangular fibrocartilage, radial portion)

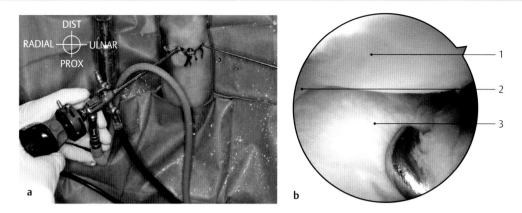

Fig. 3.35 **(a)** Right wrist with the arthroscope in portal 4–5 as the lens looks ulnar and distal. **(b)** Arthroscopic view.

1 Lunate, 2 Distal radius, 3 Articular disk (triangular fibrocartilage, radial portion)

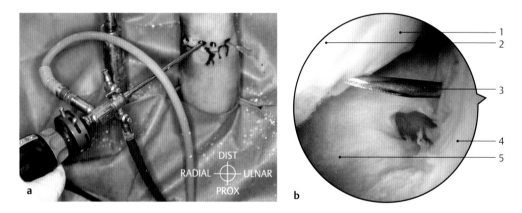

Fig. 3.36 Right wrist with the arthroscope in portal 4–5 as the lens looks ulnar for the right location of portal 6U (needle).

1 Triquetrum, 2 Lunate, 3 Portal 6U, 4 Articular disk (triangular fibrocartilage, ulnar portion), 5 Articular disk (triangular fibrocartilage, radial portion)

3.5.4 Portal 6R

Portal 6R is located between the extensor compartment 5 (extensor digiti minimi) and the extensor compartment 6 (extensor carpi ulnaris), and is always radial to the tendon extensor carpi ulnaris. This portal is useful for the evaluation of the ulnar portion of the radiocarpal joint (articular disk [triangular fibrocartilage], lunotriquetral ligament) or for instrumentation. The external anatomical landmarks are shown in **Fig. 3.37**.

Anatomy and Structures at Risk

The structures at risk are the same tendons that define the location of portal 6R, and the articular disk (triangular fibrocartilage). **Figs. 3.38–3.40** show the relevant anatomy for this portal.

Figs. 3.41–3.44 show different views of the radiocarpal joint using portal 6R.

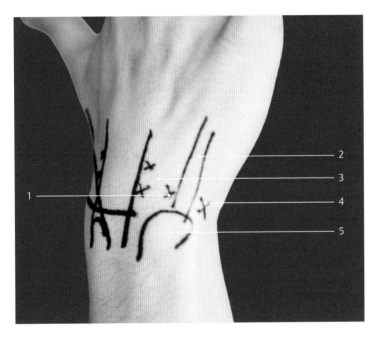

Fig. 3.37 Dorsal view of right wrist shows the external landmarks.

1 Portal 6R
2 Extensor carpi ulnaris
3 Extensor digiti minimi
4 Portal 6U
5 Distal ulna

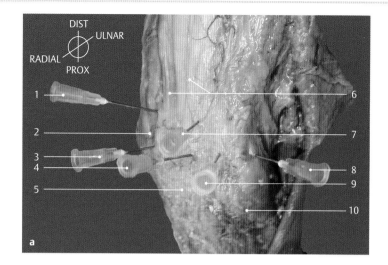

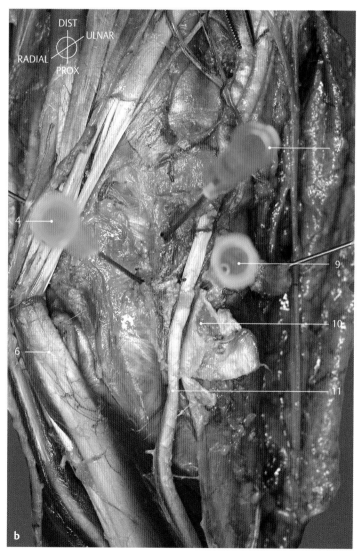

Fig. 3.38 (a, b) Dorsoulnar view of right wrist shows the location of portal 6R and the related anatomy.

1 Radial midcarpal portal
2 Extensor pollicis longus
3 Portal 3–4
4 Portal 4–5
5 Distal radius
6 Extensor digitorum
7 Ulnar midcarpal portal
8 Portal 6U
9 Portal 6 R
10 Distal ulna
11 Extensor digiti minimi

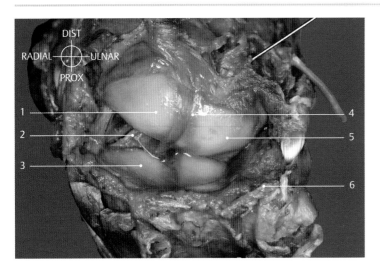

Fig. 3.39 Right wrist with the radiocarpal joint opened to show the articular structures to be examined via portal 6R.

1 Scaphoid
2 Palmar long radiolunate ligament
3 Distal radius
4 Scapholunate ligament
5 Lunate
6 Distal ulna

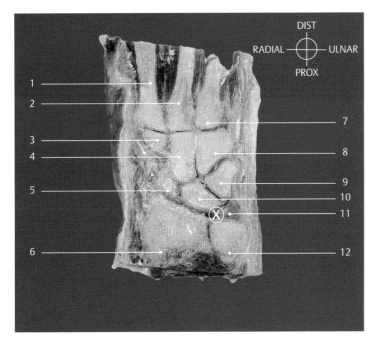

Fig. 3.40 Coronal cut that shows both carpal rows.

1 Second metacarpal bone
2 Third metacarpal bone
3 Trapezium/trapezoid
4 Capitate
5 Scaphoid
6 Distal radius
7 Fourth metacarpal bone
8 Hamate
9 Triquetrum
10 Lunate
11 Articular disk (triangular fibrocartilage)
12 Distal ulna
Ⓧ Portal 6R

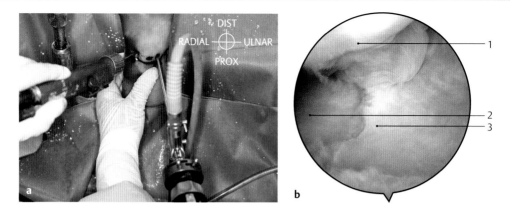

Fig. 3.41 **(a)** Right wrist with the arthroscope in portal 6R as the lens looks proximal. **(b)** Arthroscopic view.

1 Triquetrum, 2 Distal radius, 3 Articular disk (triangular fibrocartilage, radial portion)

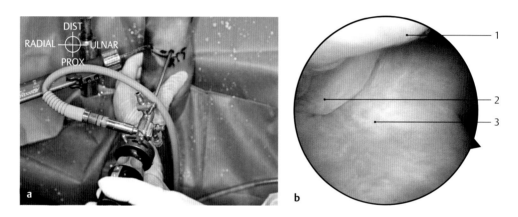

Fig. 3.42 **(a)** Right wrist with the arthroscope in portal 6R as the lens looks ulnar. **(b)** Arthroscopic view.

1 Triquetrum, 2 Distal ulna, 3 Articular disk (triangular fibrocartilage, ulnar portion)

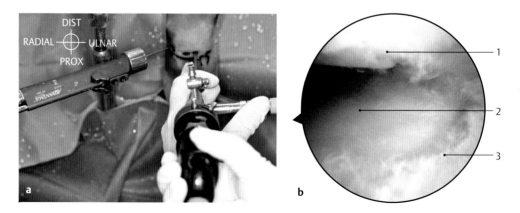

Fig. 3.43 **(a)** Right wrist with the arthroscope in portal 6R as the lens looks radial. **(b)** Arthroscopic view.

1 Lunate, 2 Distal radius, 3 Articular disk (triangular fibrocartilage, radial portion)

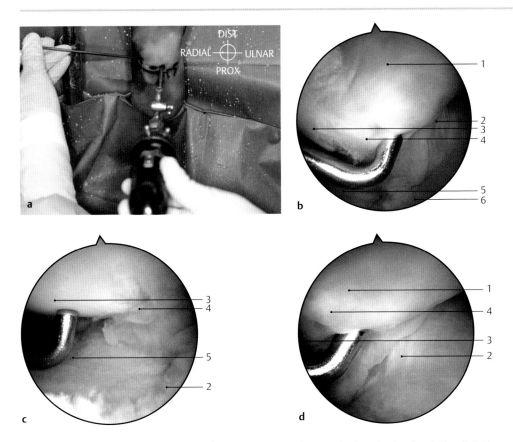

Fig. 3.44 (a) Right wrist with the arthroscope in portal 6R as the lens looks distal. **(b–d)** Arthroscopic views.

1 Triquetrum, 2 Articular disk (triangular fibrocartilage), 3 Lunate, 4 Lunotriquetral ligament, 5 Distal radius, 6 Distal ulna

3.5.5 Portal 6U

The location of portal 6U is ulnar to the extensor carpi ulnaris, between this tendon and the styloid process of the ulna. This portal is used as an instrumentation portal for lesions of the articular disk (triangular fibrocartilage). The external anatomical landmarks are shown in **Fig. 3.45**.

Anatomy and Structures at Risk

The structures at risk for portal 6U are the tendon that defines its location and the dorsal branch of the ulnar nerve. **Figs. 3.46–3.49** show the relevant anatomy of the portal. Portal 6U can be used to enter the radiocarpal joint; however, it is mainly an instrumentation portal (**Figs. 3.50 and 3.51**).

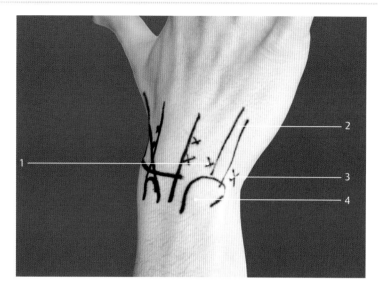

Fig. 3.45 Dorsal view of right wrist shows the external anatomical landmarks.

1 Portal 6R
2 Extensor carpi ulnaris
3 Portal 6U
4 Distal ulna

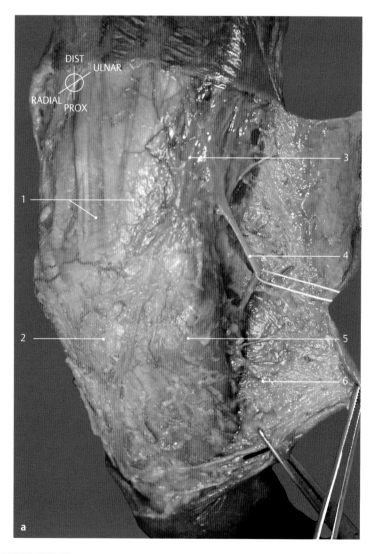

Fig. 3.46 (a, b) Dorsoulnar view of right wrist shows the dorsal branch of the ulnar nerve.

1 Extensor digitorum
2 Distal radius
3 Extensor digiti minimi
4 Dorsal branch of the ulnar nerve
5 Distal ulna
6 Skin

(Continued)

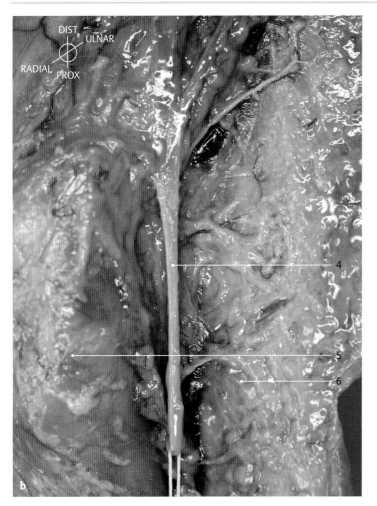

Fig. 3.46   *(continued)*
(b) Dorsoulnar view of right wrist shows the dorsal branch of the ulnar nerve.

1 Extensor digitorum
2 Distal radius
3 Extensor digiti minimi
4 Dorsal branch of the ulnar nerve
5 Distal ulna
6 Skin

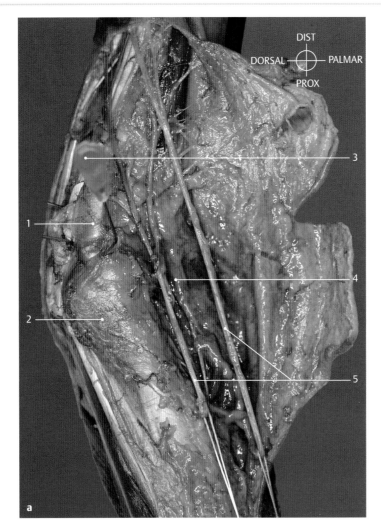

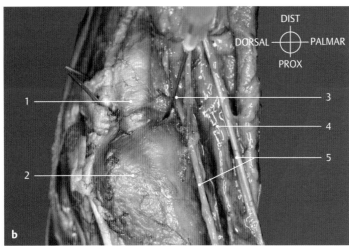

Fig. 3.47   (a, b) Ulnar view of right wrist shows the location of portal 6U and its relation to the dorsal branch of the ulnar nerve.

1 Extensor carpi ulnaris
2 Distal ulna
3 Portal 6U
4 Ulnar artery
5 Dorsal branch of the ulnar nerve (displaced)

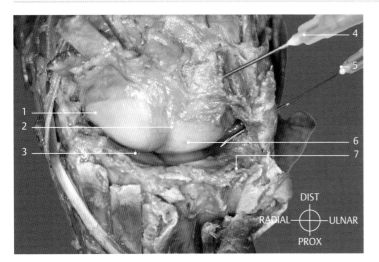

Fig. 3.48 Right wrist with the radiocarpal joint opened and the location of portal 6U marked with a needle.

1 Scaphoid
2 Scapholunate ligament
3 Distal radius
4 Ulnar midcarpal portal
5 Portal 6U
6 Lunate
7 Distal ulna

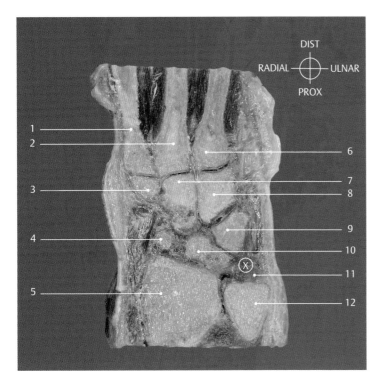

Fig. 3.49 Frontal cut of right wrist that shows the articular anatomy and the different osseous structures at the ulnar portion of the radiocarpal joint.

1 Second metacarpal bone
2 Third metacarpal bone
3 Trapezoid
4 Scaphoid
5 Distal radius
6 Fourth metacarpal bone
7 Capitate
8 Hamate
9 Triquetrum
10 Lunate
11 Articular disk (triangular fibrocartilage)
12 Distal ulna
Ⓧ Portal 6U

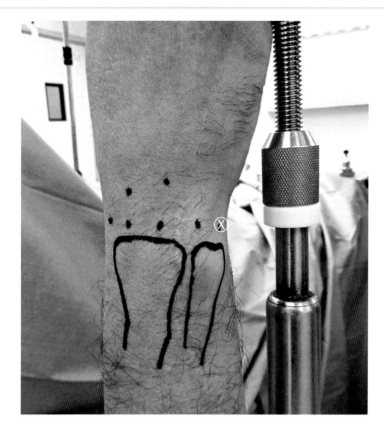

Fig. 3.50 Right wrist shows portal 6U location.
(X) Portal 6U

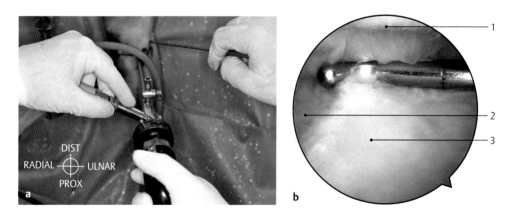

Fig. 3.51 **(a)** Right wrist with the arthroscope in portal 4–5 and the probe in portal 6U. **(b)** Arthroscopic view showing the probe in portal 6U.

1 Lunate, 2 Distal radius, 3 Articular disk (triangular fibrocartilage)

3.5.6 Radial Midcarpal Portal

The radial midcarpal portal is located 8–10 mm distal to portal 3–4 in the sulcus capitate, halfway between the base of the second metacarpal bone and the dorsal margin of the distal radius, ulnar to the extensor carpi radialis brevis tendon. This portal enters the interval between the scaphoid and the capitate. The external anatomical landmarks are shown in **Fig. 3.52.**

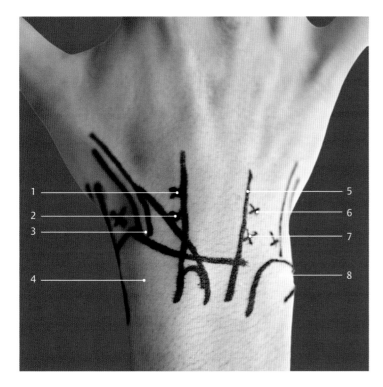

Fig. 3.52   Right wrist with the external anatomical landmarks for the radial midcarpal portal.

1 Radial midcarpal portal
2 Portal 3–4
3 Extensor carpi radiales brevis and longus
4 Distal radius
5 Extensor digitorum
6 Ulnar midcarpal portal
7 Portal 4–5
8 Distal ulna

Anatomy and Structures at Risk

The structures at risk when setting up the radial midcarpal portal are the tendons that define its location. **Figs. 3.53–3.57** show the relevant anatomy for this portal.

The interval between the scaphoid and the capitate is the working space for the radial midcarpal portal. **Figs. 3.58–3.60** show the arthroscopic anatomy for this portal.

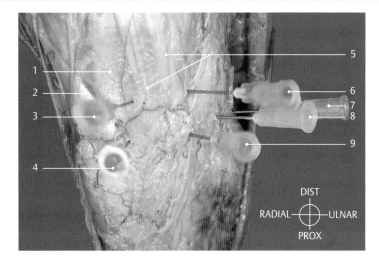

Fig. 3.53   Dorsal view of right wrist with the dorsal portals marked by needles, especially the midcarpal portals.

1 Extensor carpi radiales brevis and longus
2 Extensor pollicis longus
3 Radial midcarpal portal
4 Portal 3–4
5 Extensor digitorum
6 Ulnar midcarpal portal
7 Portal 6U
8 Portal 6R
9 Portal 4–5

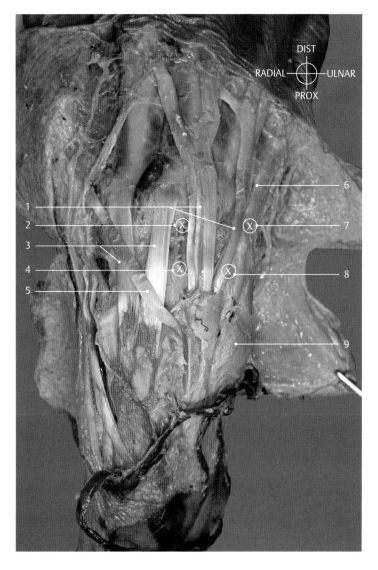

Fig. 3.54   Dorsal view of right wrist shows the tendons related to the radial midcarpal portal.

1 Extensor digitorum/extensor indicis
2 Radial midcarpal portal
3 Extensor carpi radiales brevis and longus
4 Portal 3–4
5 Extensor pollicis longus
6 Extensor digiti minimi
7 Ulnar midcarpal portal
8 Portal 4–5
9 Distal ulna

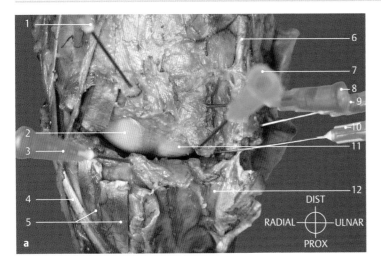

Fig. 3.55   (a) Right wrist with the radiocarpal joint opened and portals 3–4 and 4–5 marked with needles as reference for the radial and ulnar midcarpal portals, respectively. The midcarpal joint is located midway between the radiocarpal joint and the base of the metacarpal bones.

1   Radial midcarpal portal
2   Scaphoid
3   Portal 3–4
4   Extensor pollicis longus
5   Extensor carpi radiales brevis and longus
6   Extensor digiti minimi
7   Portal 4–5
8   Ulnar midcarpal portal
9   Portal 6U
10 Portal 6R
11 Lunate
12 Distal ulna

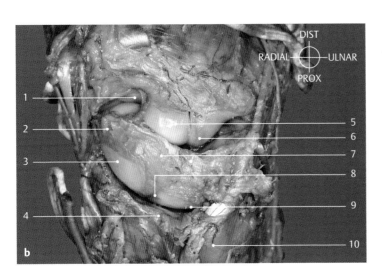

Fig. 3.55   (b) The radiocarpal joint and the midcarpal joint are opened to show the osteoarticular anatomy.

1   Trapezoid
2   Scaphotrapezio-trapezoid ligament
3   Scaphoid
4   Distal radius
5   Capitate
6   Hamate
7   Dorsal intercarpal ligament
8   Scapholunate ligament
9   Lunate
10 Distal ulna

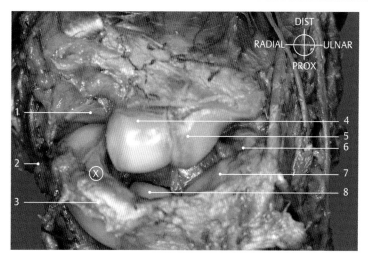

Fig. 3.56   Dorsal view of right wrist with an opened midcarpal joint.

1 Trapezoid
2 Radial artery
3 Scaphoid
4 Capitate
5 Hamate
6 Pisiformis
7 Triquetrum
8 Lunate
ⓧ Radial midcarpal portal

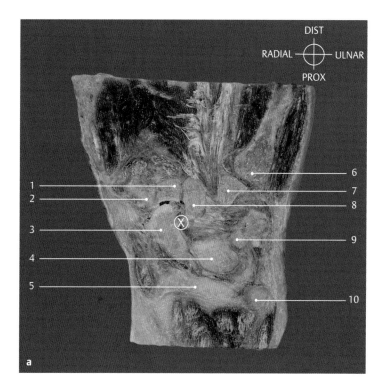

Fig. 3.57   (a, b) Frontal cuts of right wrist show the radial midcarpal joint working space between the scaphoid and the capitate.

1 Trapezoid
2 Trapezium
3 Scaphoid
4 Lunate
5 Distal radius
6 Fifth metacarpal bone
7 Hamate
8 Capitate
9 Triquetrum
10 Distal ulna
ⓧ Radial midcarpal portal

(Continued)

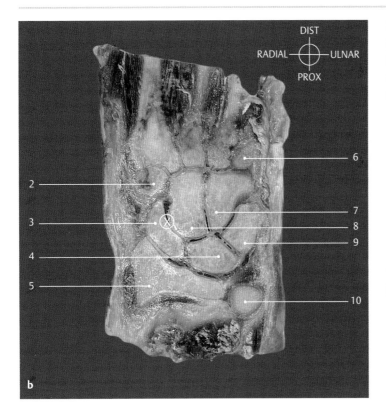

DIST
RADIAL—⊕—ULNAR
PROX

Fig. 3.57 (*continued*)
(b) Frontal cuts of right wrist show the radial midcarpal joint working space between the scaphoid and the capitate.

1 Trapezoid
2 Trapezium
3 Scaphoid
4 Lunate
5 Distal radius
6 Fifth metacarpal bone
7 Hamate
8 Capitate
9 Triquetrum
10 Distal ulna
Ⓧ Radial midcarpal portal

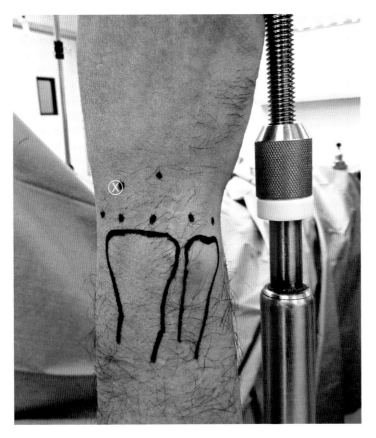

Fig. 3.58   Right wrist shows the radial midcarpal portal.
Ⓧ Radial midcarpal portal

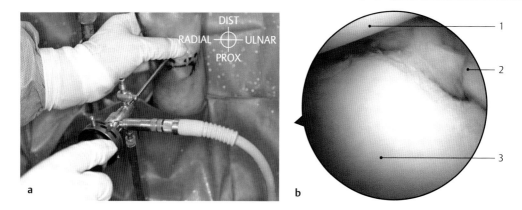

Fig. 3.59 **(a)** Right wrist with the arthroscope in the radial midcarpal portal as the lens looks radial. **(b)** Arthroscopic view.

1 Capitate, 2 Lunate, 3 Scaphoid

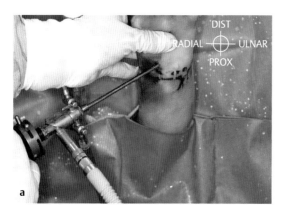

Fig. 3.60 **(a)** Right wrist with the arthroscope in the radial midcarpal portal as the lens looks dorsoradial. Minor changes in the position of the arthroscope show additional structures. **(b, c)** Arthroscopic views.

1 Capitate
2 Lunate
3 Scaphoid
4 Scapholunate ligament

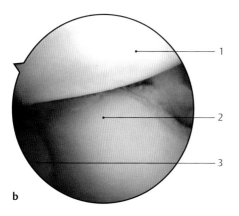

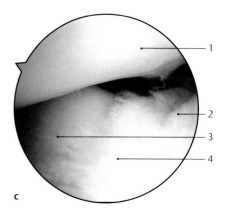

3.5.7 Ulnar Midcarpal Portal

The ulnar midcarpal portal is located distal to radiocarpal portal 4–5, in line with the fourth metacarpal bone. This portal is useful to evaluate the capitate-hamate-triquetrum-lunate interval.

It is mainly an instrumentation portal. The external anatomical landmarks are shown in **Fig. 3.61** and the anatomy and structures at risk are shown in the **Figs. 3.62–3.65. Figs. 3.66–3.70** show the arthroscopic anatomy for the ulnar midcarpal portal.

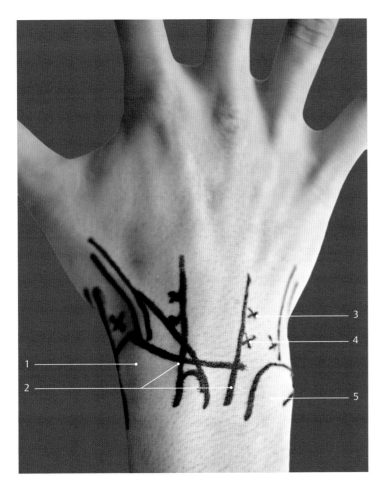

Fig. 3.61   Right wrist with the external landmarks for the ulnar midcarpal portal.

1 Distal radius
2 Extensor digitorum
3 Ulnar midcarpal portal
4 Portal 4–5
5 Distal ulna

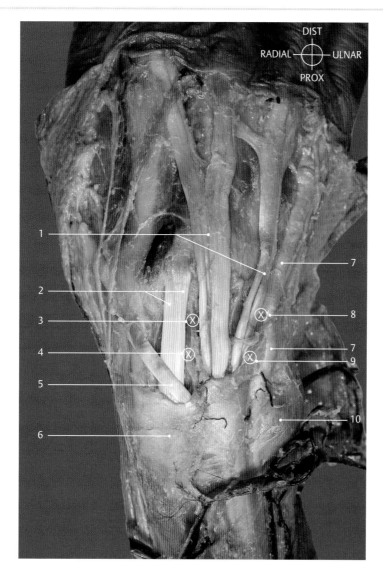

Fig. 3.62 Dorsal view of right wrist shows the tendons related to the ulnar midcarpal portal.

1 Extensor digitorum/indicis
2 Extensor carpi radiales brevis and longus
3 Radial midcarpal portal
4 Portal 3–4
5 Extensor pollicis longus
6 Extensor retinaculum-distal radius
7 Extensor digiti minimi
8 Ulnar midcarpal portal
9 Portal 4–5
10 Distal ulna

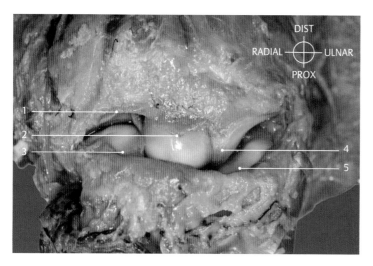

Fig. 3.63 Dorsal view of right wrist with opened midcarpal joint to evaluate the articular structures.

1 Trapezoid
2 Capitate
3 Scaphoid
4 Hamate
5 Triquetrum

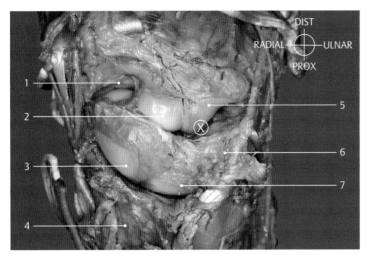

Fig. 3.64 Dorsal view of right wrist an opened radiocarpal and midcarpal joint to evaluate the articular structures.

1 Trapezoid
2 Capitate
3 Scaphoid
4 Distal radius
5 Hamate
6 Triquetrum
7 Lunate
(X) Ulnar midcarpal portal

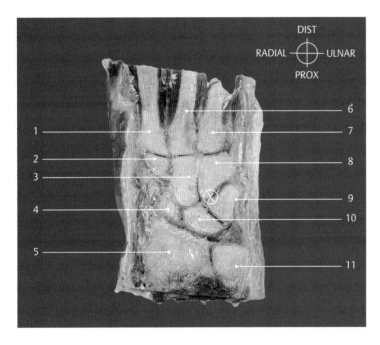

Fig. 3.65 Frontal cut of a right wrist shows the midcarpal working space (ulnar) and the capitate–hamate–triquetrum–lunate interval.

1 Second metacarpal bone
2 Trapezoid
3 Capitate
4 Scaphoid
5 Distal radius
6 Third metacarpal bone
7 Fourth metacarpal bone
8 Hamate
9 Triquetrum
10 Lunate
11 Distal ulna
(X) Ulnar midcarpal portal

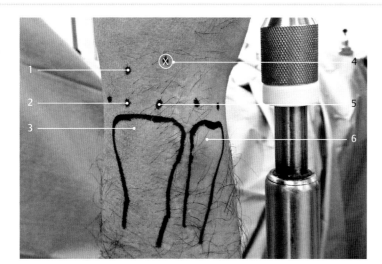

Fig. 3.66   Right wrist shows the ulnar midcarpal portal.

1 Radial midcarpal portal
2 Portal 3–4
3 Distal radius
4 Ulnar midcarpal portal
5 Portal 4–5
6 Distal ulna

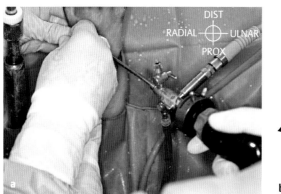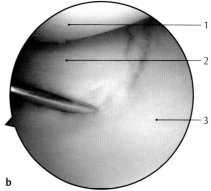

Fig. 3.67   **(a)** Right wrist with the arthroscope in the ulnar midcarpal portal as the lens looks radial. **(b)** Arthroscopic view.

1 Capitate, 2 Lunate, 3 Triquetrum

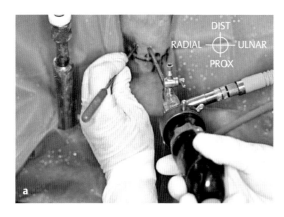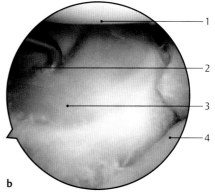

Fig. 3.68   **(a)** Right wrist with the arthroscope in the ulnar midcarpal portal as the lens looks radial for a more panoramic and ulnar view. **(b)** Arthroscopic view.

1 Capitate, 2 Scaphoid, 3 Lunate, 4 Triquetrum

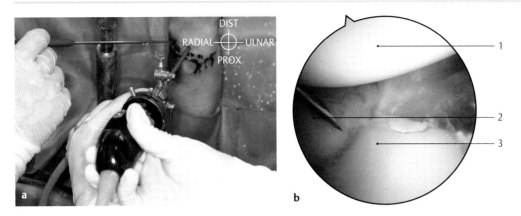

Fig. 3.69   (a) Right wrist with the arthroscope in the ulnar midcarpal portal as the lens looks distal. **(b)** Arthroscopic view.

1 Capitate, 2 Lunate, 3 Triquetrum

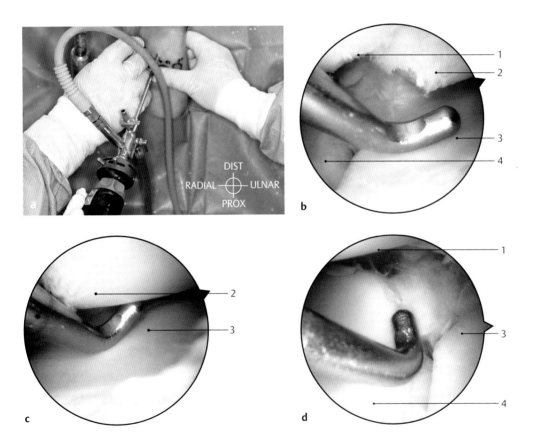

Fig. 3.70   (a) Right wrist with the arthroscope in the ulnar midcarpal portal as the lens looks ulnar and proximal. Minor changes in the position of the arthroscope show a more dorsal or palmar view of the articular structures. **(b–d)** Arthroscopic views.

1 Capitate, 2 Hamate, 3 Triquetrum, 4 Lunate

4 Hip

Cristian Blanco Moreno, Pedro Pablo Amenábar Edwards, Alejandro Zylberberg Serman, Claudio Rojas Ponce, Eduardo Leopold González, and Carlos Espech López

4.1 Introduction

Arthroscopic surgery is an important tool in the management of the painful hip. Many procedures performed previously by arthrotomy can now be accomplished using arthroscopy, with the advantages of minimally invasive surgery.

The anatomy of the hip is difficult for arthroscopic techniques and requires special equipment. The soft tissues around the hip joint, the osseous congruency, and inherent stability make access to the hip complex. The neurovascular structures around the hip joint demand an excellent knowledge of the anatomy to reduce the risk of complications during the arthroscopic procedure.

This chapter covers the positioning of the patient, the arthroscopic portals, their related anatomy, and the arthroscopic techniques used by the authors for correct visualization of the hip joint. The central and peripheral arthroscopic hip joint compartments are also discussed in terms of anatomy and arthroscopic techniques.

4.2 Anatomy

4.2.1 Extra-articular Anatomy

To get access to the hip joint it is necessary to pass through many muscular structures and close to some important neurovascular structures, as shown in **Figs. 4.1–4.5**.

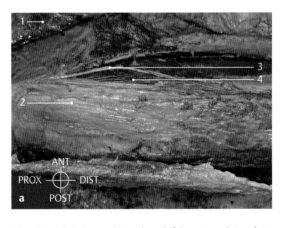
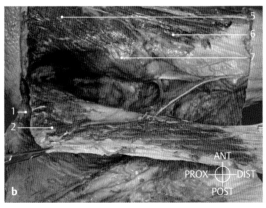

Fig. 4.1 **(a)** Anterolateral and **(b)** posterolateral views of right (cadaveric) hip.

1 Skin, 2 Iliotibial tract, 3 Lateral cutaneous nerve of the thigh, 4 Sartorius muscle, 5 Gluteus medius muscle, 6 Vastus lateralis muscle, 7 Greater trochanter

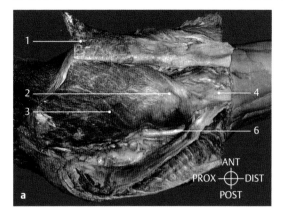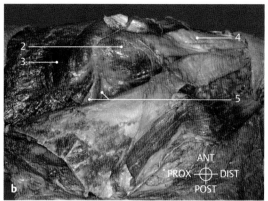

Fig. 4.2   (a) Posterolateral and **(b)** posterior view of the gluteus medius layer of right (cadaveric) hip.

1 Iliotibial tract cut, 2 Greater trochanter, 3 Gluteus medius muscle, 4 Vastus lateralis muscle,
5 External rotator muscles, 6 Sciatic nerve

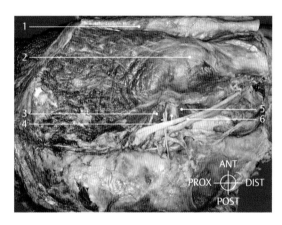

Fig. 4.3   Posterior structures of right (cadaveric) hip.

1 Iliotibial tract
2 Greater trochanter
3 Gemellus superior muscle
4 Obturator internus muscle
5 Gemellus inferior muscle
6 Sciatic nerve

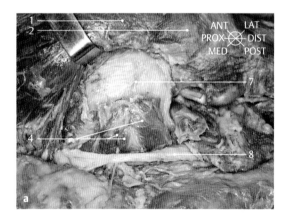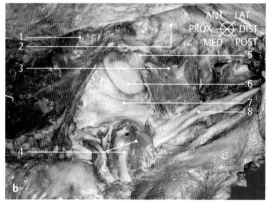

Fig. 4.4   (a, b) Posterior view of right (cadaveric) hip, with the gluteus medius and minor muscles mobilized.

1 Gluteus medius muscle, 2 Greater trochanter, 3 Quadratus femoris muscle, 4 External rotator muscles
(cut and mobilized), 5 Femoral neck, 6 Femoral head, 7 Joint capsule over femoral head, 8 Sciatic nerve

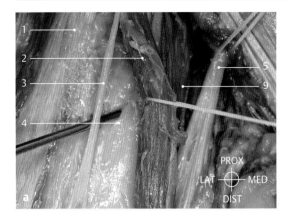

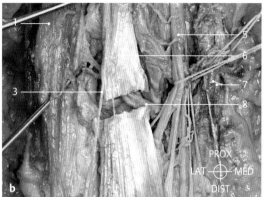

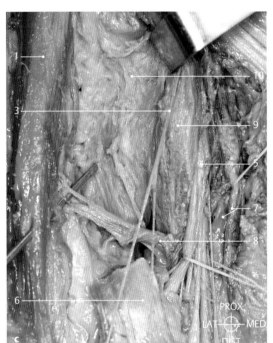

Fig. 4.5   (a–c) Close-up view of the right anterior (cadaveric) hip.

1 Tensor fasciae latae muscle
2 Sartorius muscle
3 Lateral cutaneous nerve of the thigh
4 Fat tissue over the rectus femoris muscle
5 Femoral nerve
6 Rectus femoris muscle tendon cut
7 Femoral artery and vein
8 Lateral circumflex femoral artery
9 Iliopsoas muscle
10 Hip joint capsule

4.2.2 Intra-articular Anatomy

The hip joint includes the articular surface of the acetabulum and the femoral head. The acetabulum is abducted 40 degrees in the horizontal plane and has 15 degrees of anteversion in the sagittal plane. The articular surface has a semilunar shape surrounding a central depression that lacks cartilage (acetabular fossa), which contains the pulvinar and the acetabular insertion of the ligamentum teres. Inferiorly, the acetabulum is limited by the transverse ligament. The acetabular labrum is at the periphery of the acetabular border, which has a pyramidal shape in the transverse plane. The femoral head is covered by cartilage in its medial two-thirds. At the medial part of the femoral head is a central depression called the fovea capitis where the ligamentum teres inserts. The hip is a very congruent joint because of the osseous anatomy and the acetabular labrum, as shown in **Fig. 4.6**.

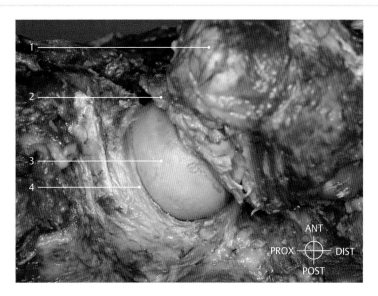

Fig. 4.6 Right (cadaveric) hip with an extensive arthrotomy showing the articular congruency of the hip joint.

1 Greater trochanter
2 Joint capsule
3 Femoral head
4 Acetabular labrum

4.3 Arthroscopic Compartments

Arthroscopic evaluation of the hip is divided into two articular compartments separated by the acetabular labrum. The central articular compartment of the hip includes all the structures deeper than the acetabular labrum, such as the acetabular fossa, the articular surface of the acetabulum, most of the articular surface of the femoral head, and the central portion of the acetabular labrum. Access to this compartment requires the use of joint distraction.

The peripheral compartment includes the femoral neck, the lateral portion of the femoral head, the retinacular vessels, the joint capsule, and the medial and lateral synovial folds. Joint distraction is not required for the evaluation of this compartment (**Figs. 4.7** and **4.8**).

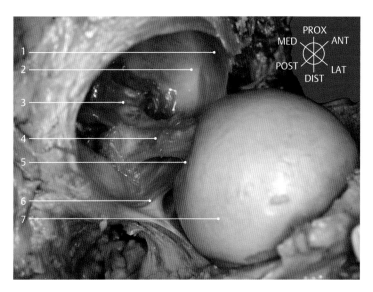

Fig. 4.7 Right (cadaveric) hip showing the structures of the central compartment.

1 Acetabular labrum
2 Acetabular cartilage
3 Pulvinar
4 Ligamentum teres
5 Fovea capitis
6 Transverse ligament
7 Femoral head

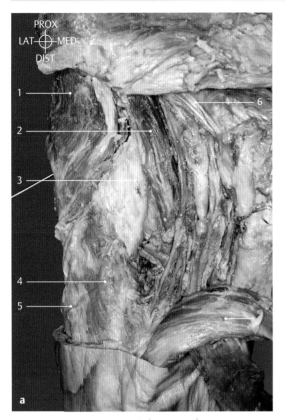

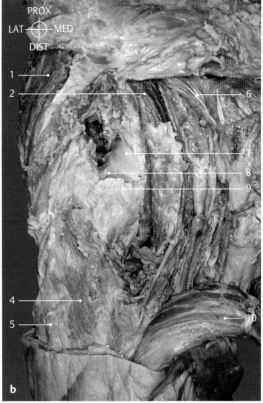

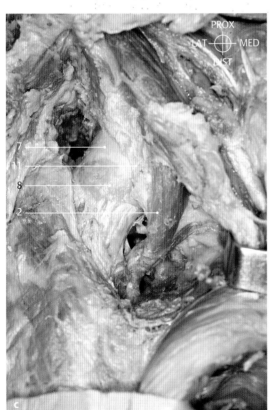

Fig. 4.8   (a–c) Frontal views of a right (cadaveric) hip showing some of the most important structures of the peripheral compartment, as well as related muscular structures.

 1 Gluteus medius muscle
 2 Iliopsoas muscle
 3 Joint capsule
 4 Vastus intermedius muscle
 5 Vastus lateralis muscle
 6 Inguinal ligament
 7 Femoral head
 8 Femoral neck
 9 Joint capsule (opened)
10 Rectus femoris muscle
11 Acetabular labrum

4.4 Pathologies Treated by Hip Arthroscopy

The indications for a hip arthroscopy are:

- Femoroacetabular impingement in its different types
- Isolated lesions of the acetabular labrum
- Septic arthritis
- Intra-articular loose bodies
- Intra-articular biopsy procedures
- Synovial pathology

4.5 Patient Positioning

Hip arthroscopy, with or without distraction, can be performed in the lateral decubitus or supine positions. The authors of this chapter suggest the supine position, as described here.

The patient is placed on the traction table and the padded perineal post is lateralized toward the site of surgery, with the hip flexed 20 degrees and the foot internally rotated 30 degrees. Once the patient is in place, traction is applied until a joint distraction of 1 cm is achieved and confirmed by fluoroscopy (**Fig. 4.9**).

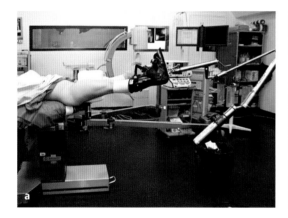

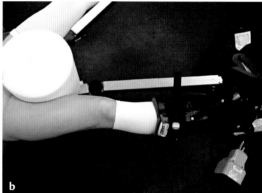

Fig. 4.9 **(a, b)** Patient positioning for arthroscopy of the right hip. **(c)** Fluoroscopic view of the distraction.

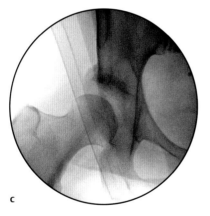

4.6 Arthroscopic Portals

Many different portals have been described for hip arthroscopy; however, depending on the pathology to be treated, two or three portals should be enough for a complete arthroscopic evaluation of the hip. The paratrochanteric anterolateral, the paratrochanteric posterolateral, and the mid anterior portals are the most frequently used (**Fig. 4.10**).

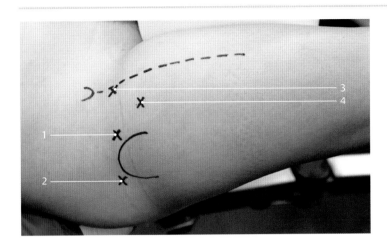

Fig. 4.10 The most frequently used arthroscopic portals for hip arthroscopy.

1 Paratrochanteric anterolateral portal
2 Paratrochanteric posterolateral portal
3 Anterior portal
4 Mid anterior portal

4.6.1 Anterolateral Paratrochanteric Portal

The anterolateral paratrochanteric portal is the first portal to be established; therefore, the use of fluoroscopy is mandatory (**Fig. 4.11a**). The remaining portals can be established under direct arthroscopic control. The anterolateral paratrochanteric portal is located 1 cm anterior to the tip of the trochanter, aiming 10 to 20 degrees cephalic and 20 to 30 degrees posterior (**Figs. 4.11 (b–d)–4.12**).

Structures at Risk

The structure at risk when using the paratrochanteric anterolateral portal is the superior gluteus nerve: after leaving the major sciatic notch, it runs transversely posterior to anterior over the deep surface of the gluteus medius muscle (**Fig. 4.13**).

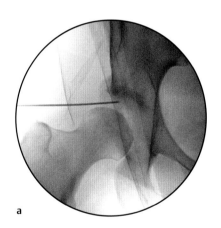

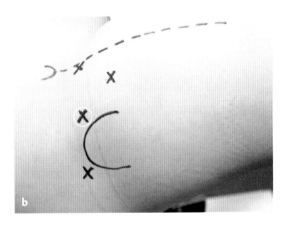

Fig. 4.11 (a) Fluoroscopic view. (b–d) Placement of the anterolateral portal in right hip. (*Continued*)

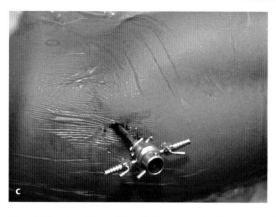
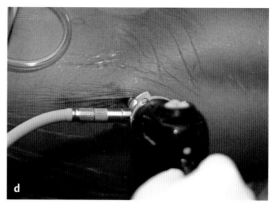

Fig. 4.11 (*continued*) **(c, d)** Placement of the anterolateral portal in right hip.

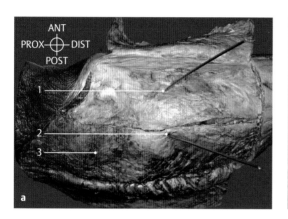
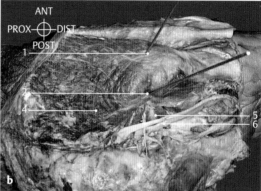

Fig. 4.12 **(a, b)** Right (cadaveric) hip showing the paratrochanteric anterolateral and posterolateral portals marked with Steinmann rods.

1 Anterolateral paratrochanteric portal, 2 Posterolateral paratrochanteric portal, 3 Gluteus major muscle, 4 Gluteus medius muscle, 5 External rotator muscle of the hip, 6 Sciatic nerve

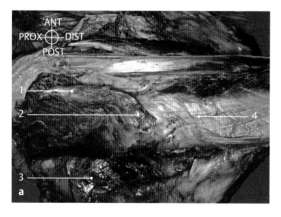
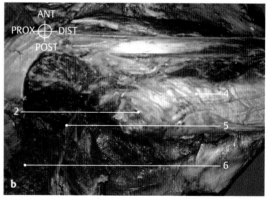

Fig. 4.13 **(a, b)** Right (cadaveric) hip shows the gluteus medius muscle layer; once mobilized, its deeper surface is visualized.

1 Gluteus medius muscle, 2 Greater trochanter, 3 Gluteus major muscle retracted, 4 Vastus lateralis muscle, 5 Superior gluteus neurovascular bundle, 6 Gluteus medius muscle mobilized posteriorly

4.6.2 Posterolateral Paratrochanteric Portal

The posterolateral paratrochanteric portal is located 1 cm posterior to the tip of the greater trochanter, directed 10 degrees proximal and 30 degrees anterior (**Fig. 4.14**). It passes through the gluteus medius and gluteus minor muscles before entering the posterior hip joint capsule (**Figs. 4.15** and **4.16**). The posterolateral paratrochanteric portal is used less frequently—its benefits can be seen in posterior lesions of the labrum and posteriorly migrated loose bodies.

Structures at Risk

The structures at risk when using the posterolateral paratrochanteric portal are the sciatic nerve at the level of the joint capsule and the superior gluteal nerve (**Fig. 4.17**).

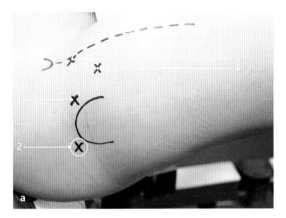

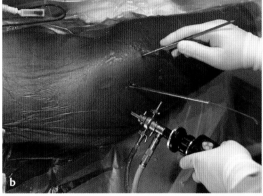

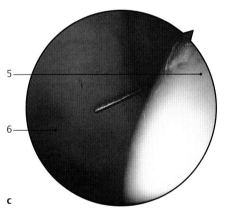

Fig. 4.14   (a, b) Right hip shows the location of the posterolateral paratrochanteric portal. **(c)** Arthroscopic view.

1 Anterolateral paratrochanteric portal
2 Posterolateral paratrochanteric portal
3 Anterior portal
4 Mid anterior portal
5 Femoral head
6 Posterior acetabulum

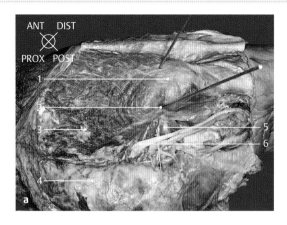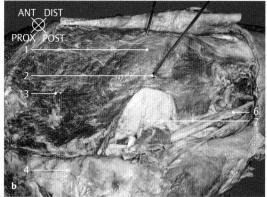

Fig. 4.15   (a, b) Right (cadaveric) hip showing the location of the posterolateral paratrochanteric portal and related structures.

1 Greater trochanter, 2 Posterolateral paratrochanteric portal, 3 Gluteus medius muscle,
4 Gluteus major muscle mobilized, 5 External rotator muscles, 6 Sciatic nerve,
7 Hip joint capsule

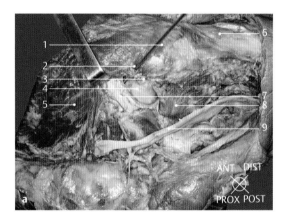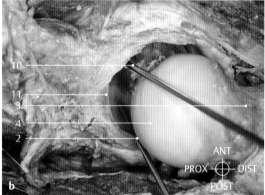

Fig. 4.16   (a, b) Right (cadaveric) hip showing the paratrochanteric posterolateral portal and the hip joint entering point, after passing through the gluteus medius and minor muscles.

1 Greater trochanter, 2 Posterolateral paratrochanteric portal, 3 Femoral neck,
4 Femoral head, 5 Gluteus medius muscle, 6 Vastus lateralis muscle,
7 Hip joint capsule opened and external rotator muscles mobilized, 8 Quadratus femoris muscle,
9 Sciatic nerve, 10 Anterolateral paratrochanteric portal, 11 Acetabular labrum

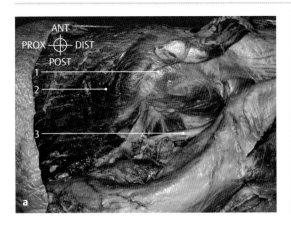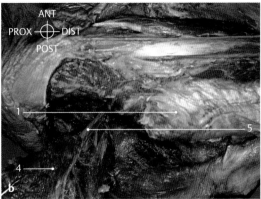

Fig. 4.17 (a, b) Right (cadaveric) hip showing the structures at risk when utilizing the posterolateral paratrochanteric portal.

1 Greater trochanter, 2 Gluteus medius muscle, 3 Sciatic nerve, 4 Gluteus medius muscle posteriorly mobilized, 5 Superior gluteal neurovascular bundle

4.6.3 Mid Anterior Portal

The mid anterior portal is located at the apex of an equilateral triangle; the base of this triangle is a line between the anterolateral paratrochanteric portal and the anterior portal. The instruments are oriented 15 degrees proximally and 20 degrees posteriorly (**Figs. 4.18** and **4.19**). This portal passes through the tensor fasciae latae muscle and penetrates the interval between the gluteus minor muscle and the rectus femoris muscle (**Fig. 4.20**).

Structures at Risk

The structures at risk when using the mid anterior portal are the lateral cutaneous nerve of the thigh and the ascending branch of the femoral circumflex artery. The lateral cutaneous nerve of the thigh divides into three or more branches at the level of the anterior portal and one of these branches may be damaged when establishing the mid anterior portal (**Fig. 4.21**). The position of the ascending branch of the femoral circumflex artery is variable but usually can be found 3 to 4 cm below the level of the anterior portal and is even closer to the mid anterior portal (**Fig. 4.22**).

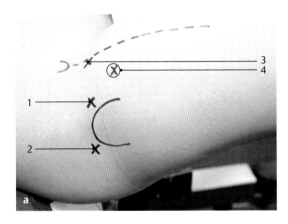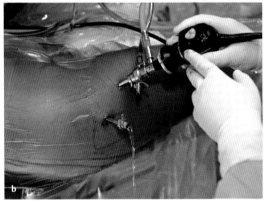

Fig. 4.18 (a, b) Right (cadaveric) hip showing the location of the arthroscope in the mid anterior portal.

1 Anterolateral paratrochanteric portal, 2 Posterolateral paratrochanteric portal, 3 Anterior portal, 4 Mid anterior portal

113

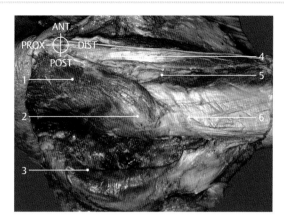

Fig. 4.19 Right (cadaveric) hip showing some of the muscular structures related to the mid anterior portal.

1 Gluteus medius muscle
2 Greater trochanter
3 Gluteus major muscle mobilized
4 Tensor fasciae latae muscle
5 Rectus femoris muscle
6 Vastus lateralis muscle

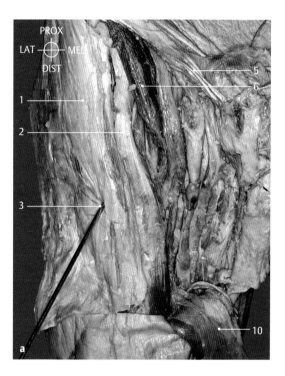
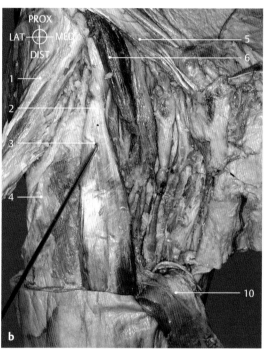

Fig. 4.20 (a, b) Frontal views of right (cadaveric) hip. The mid anterior portal is marked with a trocar over the tensor fasciae latae muscle, close to its limit with the rectus femoris muscle. The muscular layers are sequentially dissected to get access to the hip joint.

1 Tensor fasciae latae muscle, 2 Rectus femoris muscle, 3 Mid anterior portal, 4 Vastus lateralis muscle,
5 Inguinal ligament, 6 Iliopsoas muscle, 7 Hip joint capsule (cut in **d**), 8 Femoral head,
9 Femoral neck, 10 Sartorius muscle

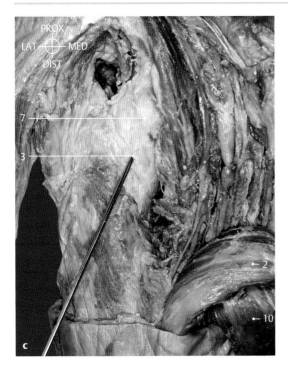

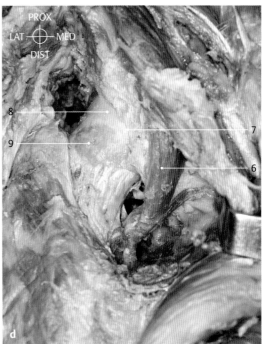

Fig. 4.20   (*continued*) **(c, d)** Frontal views of right (cadaveric) hip. The mid anterior portal is marked with a trocar over the tensor fasciae latae muscle, close to its limit with the rectus femoris muscle. The muscular layers are sequentially dissected to get access to the hip joint.

1 Tensor fasciae latae muscle, 2 Rectus femoris muscle, 3 Mid anterior portal, 4 Vastus lateralis muscle, 5 Inguinal ligament, 6 Iliopsoas muscle, 7 Hip joint capsule (cut in **d**), 8 Femoral head, 9 Femoral neck, 10 Sartorius muscle

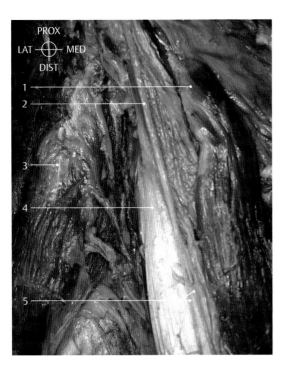

Fig. 4.21   Right (cadaveric) hip showing the femoral cutaneous nerve of the thigh and its branches.

1 Sartorius muscle
2 Lateral cutaneous nerve of the thigh
3 Gluteus medius muscle
4 Tensor fasciae latae muscle
5 Branches of the lateral
    cutaneous nerve of the thigh

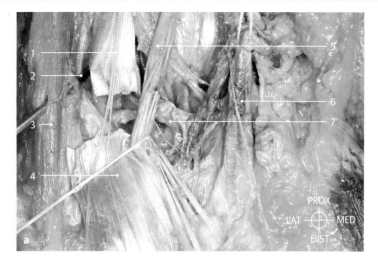

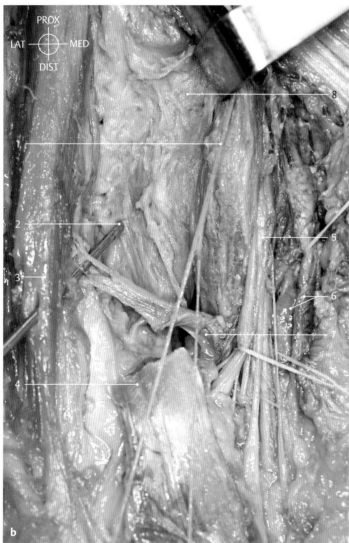

Fig. 4.22 (a, b) Right (cadaveric) hip showing the mid anterior portal marked by a Steinmann rod. The anatomical structures related to the mid anterior portal are also shown.

1 Lateral cutaneous nerve of the thigh
2 Mid anterior portal
3 Tensor fasciae latae muscle
4 Rectus femoris muscle (cut)
5 Femoral nerve
6 Femoral artery and vein
7 Ascending branch of the circumflex femoral artery
8 Hip joint capsule

4.6.4 Anterior Portal

The anterior portal is located at the intersection between one vertical line running distally from the anterior iliac spine (AIS) and a second horizontal line running transversely at the level of the tip of the greater trochanter, 4 to 6 cm distal to the AIS (**Fig. 4.23**). The trocar should be directed 30 degrees medially and 45 degrees proximally. This portal passes through the sartorius and rectus femoris muscles before reaching the hip joint capsule (**Fig. 4.24**). It is a portal that is used less frequently because its benefits are well covered by the mid anterior portal.

Structures at Risk

The structures at risk when using the anterior portal are similar as for the mid anterior portal. They are the lateral cutaneous nerve of the thigh, the femoral nerve, and the ascending branch of the circumflex femoral artery (**Fig. 4.24**).

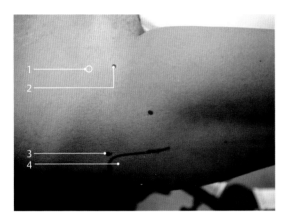

Fig. 4.23 Right hip in the supine position showing the anatomical landmarks and location of the anterior portal.

1 Anterosuperior iliac spine
2 Anterior portal
3 Anterior paratrochanteric portal
4 Tip of the greater trochanter

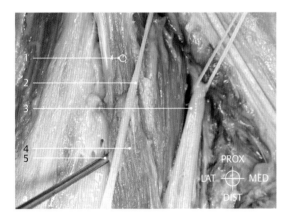
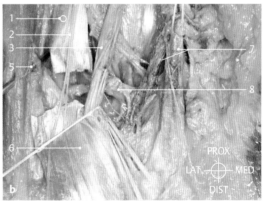

Fig. 4.24 (a, b) Anterior view of right (cadaveric) hip showing the related anatomical structures at risk when using the anterior portal.

1 Anterior portal, 2 Lateral cutaneous nerve of the thigh, 3 Femoral nerve, 4 Sartorius muscle, 5 Mid anterior portal, 6 Rectus femoris muscle, 7 Femoral artery and vein, 8 Ascending branch of the femoral circumflex artery

4.7   Suggested Sequence for a Diagnostic Arthroscopy of the Central Compartment

A complete arthroscopic evaluation of the hip uses at least two portals. For an evaluation of the central compartment a 70-degree lens is necessary. The acetabular labrum, the periphery of the articular surface of the acetabulum, and the central part of the femoral head are visualized during the procedure.

For descriptive and orientation purposes, the articular surface of the labrum can be seen as a watch, with the 12 o'clock position being the most superior point (the stellar sign) and the 6 o'clock position the most inferior point (the transverse ligament). In the case of a right hip, the 9 o'clock position represents the posterior wall of the acetabulum and the 3 o'clock position is the anterior wall (for the left hip, it is the opposite).

The following arthroscopic description uses the anterolateral paratrochanteric portal as the initial portal and the suggested sequence is shown in **Figs. 4.25–4.36**.

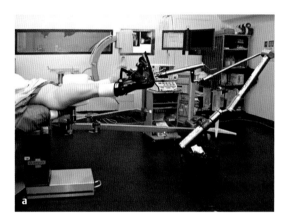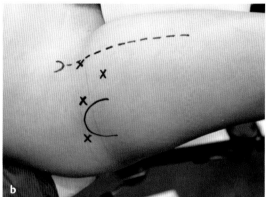

Fig. 4.25   (a) As described previously for arthroscopic surgery of the right hip, the patient is supine with anatomical landmarks noted. **(b)** Anatomical landmarks have been noted on the right hip as the patient lies in supine position.

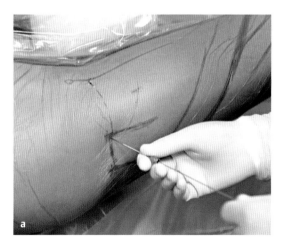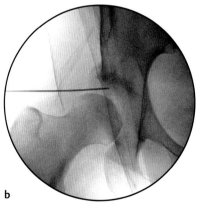

Fig. 4.26   (a) The required distraction is applied and the location of the anterolateral paratrochanteric portal is checked by fluoroscopy. **(b)** Fluoroscopic view.

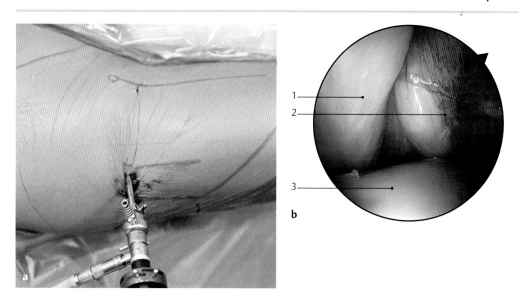

Fig. 4.27   (a) The 70-degree arthroscope in the anterolateral paratrochanteric portal shows the anterior security triangle (the lens looks distally and anterior). **(b)** Arthroscopic view.

1 Acetabular labrum, 2   Hip joint capsule (anterior security triangle), 3 Femoral head

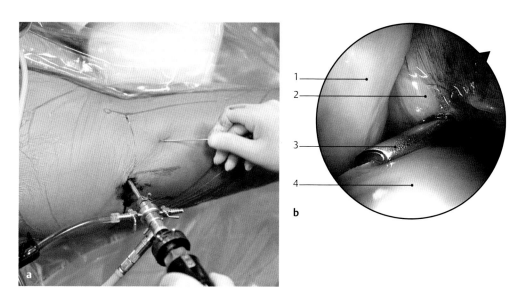

Fig. 4.28   (a) The 70-degree arthroscope is in the anterolateral paratrochanteric portal and shows the instrumentation through the anterior security triangle to locate the mid anterior portal. The lens looks distally and anterior. **(b)** Arthroscopic view.

1 Acetabular labrum, 2 Hip joint capsule (anterior security triangle), 3 Spinal needle through the joint capsule, 4 Femoral head

119

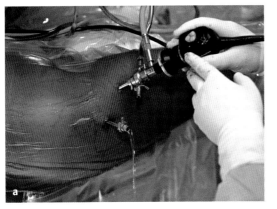 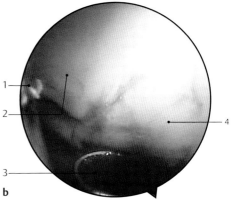

Fig. 4.29 **(a)** The arthroscope is moved to the mid anterior portal and the lens looks posteriorly to visualize the posterior security triangle. It is important to note that when you switch the arthroscope to the mid anterior portal the view is a mirror image of the one obtained before, so the femoral head is now on the left and the acetabulum is on the right. **(b)** Arthroscopic view.

1 Femoral head, 2 Semilunar cartilage, 3 Arthroscopic cannula entering the joint through the anterolateral paratrochanteric portal, 4 Acetabular labrum

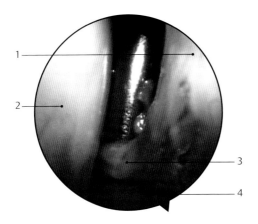

Fig. 4.30 The arthroscope is in the mid anterior portal to control the position of the instrument introduced into the joint via the anterolateral paratrochanteric portal. In the case of an unexpected labrum penetration, the arthroscope should be relocated under direct arthroscopic control using the mid anterior portal. Arthroscopic view showing the instrument through the labrum.

1 Acetabular labrum
2 Femoral head
3 Cannula through the labrum
4 Joint capsule

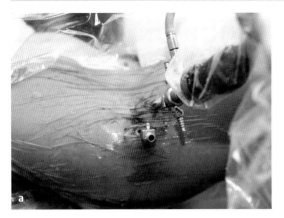

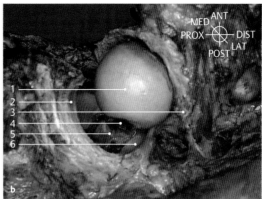

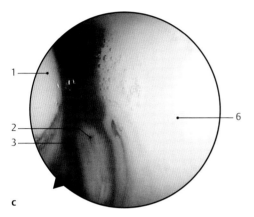

Fig. 4.31 (a–c) Arthroscope in the mid anterior portal of the right hip is driven to the fovea capitis—the lens looks posteriorly. The anatomical and arthroscopic views are shown.

1 Femoral head
2 Acetabular labrum 9 o'clock to 11 o'clock
3 Joint capsule
4 Fovea capitis
5 Ligament of the femoral head
6 Semilunar cartilage of the acetabulum

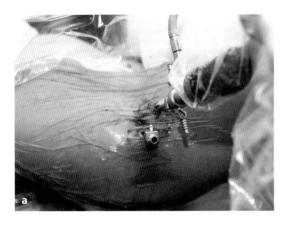

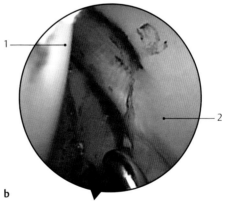

Fig. 4.32 (a) The arthroscope remains in the mid anterior portal and is moved to a more superficial point than the previous position. The lens looks posterior to evaluate the anterior acetabular labrum.
(b) Arthroscopic view.

1 Femoral head, 2 Acetabular labrum (1 o'clock to 3 o'clock)

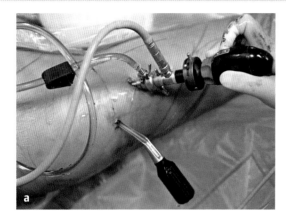

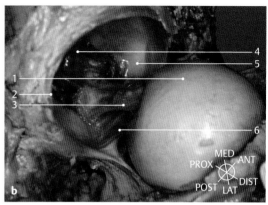

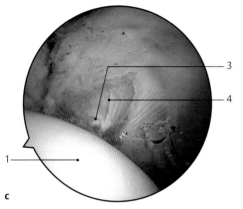

Fig. 4.33 (a–c) The arthroscope remains in the mid anterior portal, and the lens looks posterior to evaluate the ligamentum teres. Anatomical and arthroscopic views.

1 Femoral head
2 Acetabular labrum
3 Ligamentum teres
4 Pulvinar
5 Acetabular semilunar cartilage
6 Transverse ligament

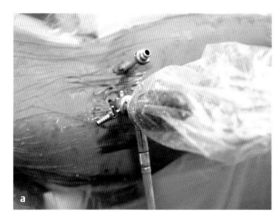

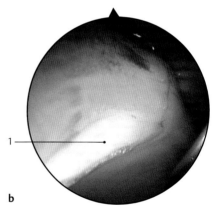

Fig. 4.34 (a) The arthroscope is switched to the anterolateral paratrochanteric portal and the lens is rotated to look anterior to evaluate the anterior labrum. The arthroscope is moved to a more superficial position. **(b)** Arthroscopic view.

1 Acetabular labrum (11 o'clock to 1 o'clock)

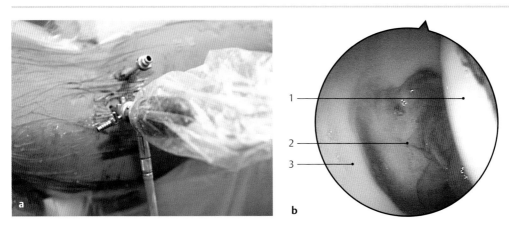

Fig. 4.35   (a) Evaluation of the pulvinar and the semilunar cartilage of the acetabulum. The arthroscope is located in the anterolateral paratrochanteric portal and the lens looks anterior. **(b)** Arthroscopic view.

1 Femoral head, 2 Pulvinar, 3 Articular cartilage of the acetabulum (semilunar)

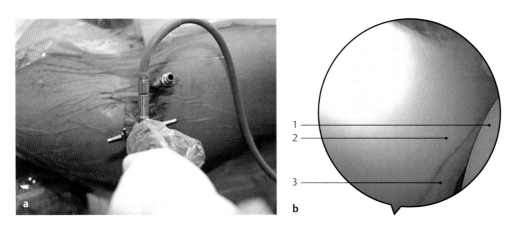

Fig. 4.36   (a) Evaluation of the final part of the semilunar cartilage of the acetabulum. The arthroscope is in the anterolateral paratrochanteric portal and the lens looks posterior. **(b)** Arthroscopic view.

1 Femoral head, 2 Articular cartilage of the acetabulum (posterolateral), 3 Acetabular labrum

4.8   Suggested Sequence for a Diagnostic Arthroscopy of the Peripheral Compartment

To perform a thorough arthroscopic evaluation of the peripheral compartment of the hip, it is necessary to control the degree of traction, the rotation of the lens, and the different positions of the hip joint (flexion, extension, abduction, adduction, and ro-

tation). It is necessary to release the limb from the traction table or to use a special pneumatic limb positioning device.

The arthroscopic evaluation starts with the arthroscope in the mid anterior portal or in the anterolateral paratrochanteric portal. The mid anterior portal is useful when evaluating the anteromedial portion of the femoral head whereas the anterolateral paratrochanteric portal is useful when evaluating the superolateral part of the femoral head. The authors use the anterolateral paratrochanteric portal as the starting portal to evaluate the peripheral compartment of the hip.

The arthroscope is removed from the central compartment of the hip and is positioned at the level of the anterior part of the femoral head—lat-er it is aimed toward the femoral neck. The joint capsule covering the femoral head–neck junction is resected (the femoral deformity causing femoroacetabular impingement is located at this level) (**Figs. 4.37–4.40**).

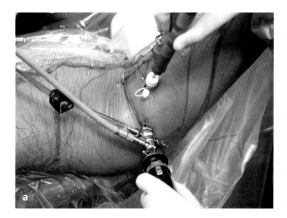

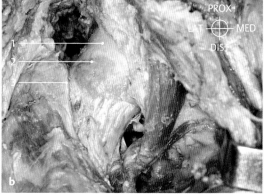

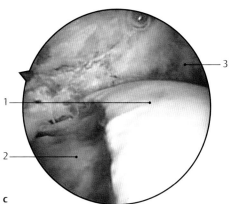

Fig. 4.37   (a) The traction is released, the right hip is flexed to 45 degrees, the arthroscope is in the anterolateral paratrochanteric portal, and the lens looks toward the femoral neck. The arthroscopic view shows the head–neck junction and the cadaveric hip dissection shows the same structures.

(b) Anatomical view. **(c)** Arthroscopic view.

1 Femoral head
2 Femoral neck
3 Hip joint capsule

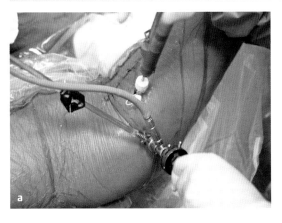

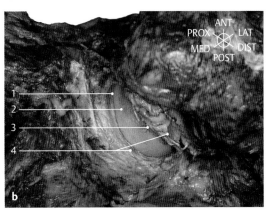

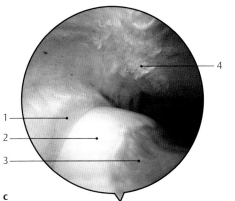

Fig. 4.38 **(a)** Arthroscopic control of the restitution of the hip articular congruency. The arthroscope remains in the anterolateral paratrochanteric portal and is moved toward the acetabulum with the lens still looking posterior. The traction is completely released and the articular congruency is checked under direct arthroscopic control. **(b)** The anatomical dissection of a right cadaveric hip shows the same articular congruency. **(c)** Arthroscopic view.

1 Acetabular labrum
2 Femoral head
3 Femoral neck
4 Hip joint capsule

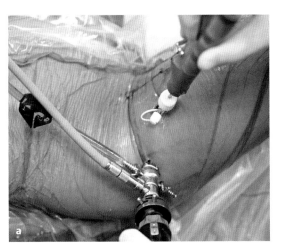

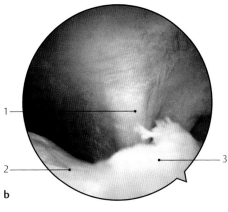

Fig. 4.39 **(a)** Evaluation of the orbicular ligament and the medial synovial fold. With 45 degrees of hip flexion, the arthroscope is driven inferiorly, the lens looks posterior distal, and the orbicularis ligament and the medial synovial fold are identified. **(b)** Arthroscopic view.

1 Orbicularis ligament, 2 Femoral neck, 3 Medial synovial fold

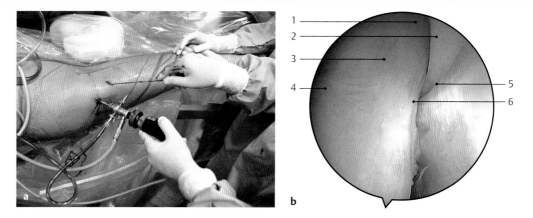

Fig. 4.40 **(a)** Evaluation of the lateral region of the hip. The hip is put back to its initial arthroscopic position in extension. The arthroscope is in the anterolateral paratrochanteric portal to check the lateral region of the head–neck junction. The lateral synovial fold and the entry of the retinacular vessels that irrigate the femoral head are in this region. **(b)** Arthroscopic view.

1 Femoral head, 2 Acetabular labrum, 3 Retinacular vessels toward the femoral head, 4 Femoral neck, 5 Orbicularis zone, 6 Lateral synovial fold

5 Knee

Cristian Blanco Moreno, Eduardo Vega Pizarro, and Juan Pablo Quinteros Pomar

5.1 Introduction

The knee is one of the joints most frequently treated with arthroscopy. A detailed knowledge of the anatomy of this joint is indispensable given the high number, diversity, and complexity of knee pathologies that can be treated with arthroscopic techniques. The anatomical relation between the portals and the knee's anatomical structures—especially neurovascular structures—is very important to note so as to avoid complications caused by the arthroscopic instrumentation.

This chapter analyzes the anterior approach with anteromedial and anterolateral portals, along with the posterior approach with posteromedial and posterolateral portals. For each portal, the external anatomical landmarks, the arthroscopic view from that specific portal, and the related anatomy are shown. Other optional portals are briefly mentioned.

5.2 Patient Positioning

The position of the patient depends on the surgeon's preference and the pathology to be treated. Routine arthroscopic procedures can be performed easily on a conventional table with the patient placed supine and the limb angled off the lateral aspect of the table. A lateral post is useful to apply valgus force to the leg. Our preference is to place the patient on the table with a leg holder, just as in the **Fig. 5.1**.

5.3 Portals

5.3.1 Anterior Portals

The anteromedial and anterolateral portals are the standard portals for the majority of arthroscopic procedures of the knee.

Anterolateral Portal

The anterolateral portal is the standard for diagnostic arthroscopy of the knee. It is located 1 cm above the lateral joint line and 1 cm lateral to the margin of the patellar ligament (**Fig. 5.2**).

Anteromedial Portal

The anteromedial portal is the initial portal during knee arthroscopy. The final location of this portal depends on the procedure and the correct placement is checked under direct arthroscopic control. In general, the anteromedial portal is located 1 cm above the medial joint line and 1 cm medial to the margin of the patellar ligament (**Fig. 5.3**).

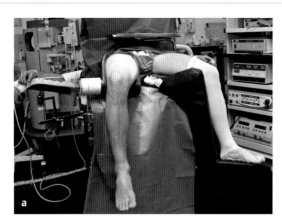

Fig. 5.1 **(a, b)** Patient in supine position on the table. Notice the use of a leg holder.

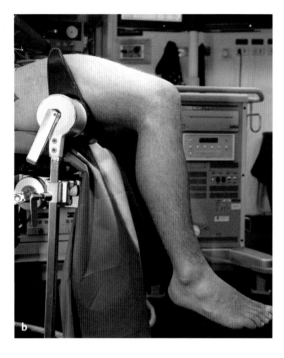

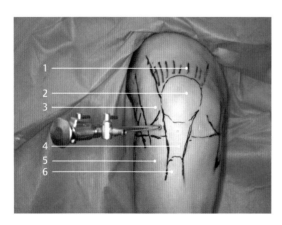

Fig. 5.2 Anterior view of right knee flexed to 90 degrees; the arthroscopic cannula is inserted via the anterolateral portal. The key anatomical landmarks are shown.

1 Quadriceps muscle tendon
2 Patella
3 Lateral femoral condyle
4 Patellar ligament
5 Lateral tibial condyle
6 Tibial tuberosity

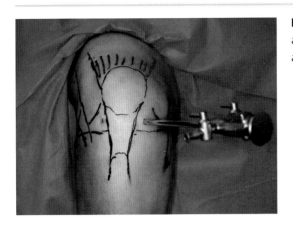

Fig. 5.3 Arthroscopic cannula is inserted via the anteromedial portal. The key anatomical landmarks are shown.

5.3.2 Posterior Portals

Posterior portals are used less frequently but are very useful when addressing complex lesions of the knee. The related anatomical structures are relevant and analyzed later in this chapter.

Posteromedial Portal

The posteromedial portal is located in a triangular soft spot formed by the posteromedial edge of the femoral condyle and the proximal tibia, 1 cm above the joint line. The knee must be flexed to 90 degrees to locate the portal behind the medial collateral ligament and anterior to the semimembranosus muscle tendon (**Fig. 5.4**).

Posterolateral Portal

The posterolateral portal is located at the intersection of the posterior femoral shaft line and a line drawn along the posterior margin of the fibula: 2 cm above the joint line, posterior to the iliotibial tract, and anterior to the biceps femoris muscle tendon. The knee must be flexed to 90 degrees (**Fig. 5.5**).

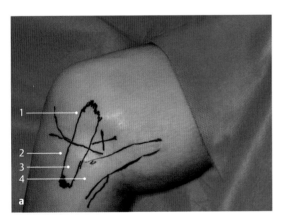

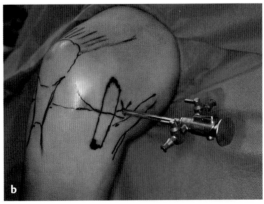

Fig 5.4 **(a)** Medial view of right knee flexed to 90 degrees, which is important to protect the posterior neurovascular structures and help the instrumentation by relaxing the posteromedial tissues. The anatomical landmarks and the location of the posteromedial portal (marked with an X) are shown. **(b)** Right knee with the arthroscopic cannula in the posteromedial portal.

1 Medial femoral condyle, 2 Medial tibial condyle, 3 Medial collateral ligament, 4 Semimembranosus muscle tendon

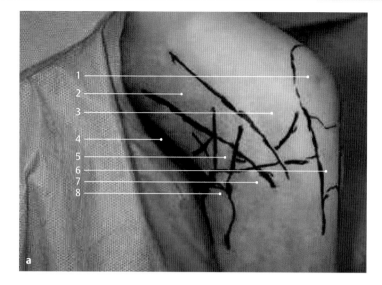

Fig. 5.5 (a) Right knee flexed to 90 degrees with lateral and posterolateral landmarks. The location of the posterolateral portal is marked with an X. **(b)** Lateral view of right knee with the arthroscopic cannula in the posterolateral portal.

1 Patella
2 Iliotibial tract
3 Lateral femoral condyle
4 Biceps femoris muscle tendon
5 Lateral collateral ligament
6 Patellar ligament
7 Lateral tibial condyle
8 Fibula

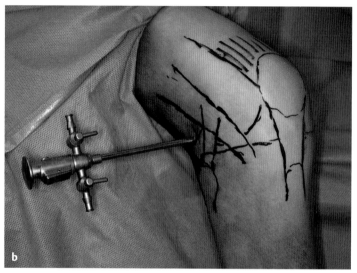

5.3.3 Accessory Portals

The following accessory portals are clinically relevant but less complex from an anatomical point of view:

- Central transpatellar ligament portal (**Fig. 5.6**)
- Superolateral portal (**Figs. 5.7**)
- Superomedial portal (**Fig. 5.8**)

5.4   Arthroscopy of the Knee: Anterior

The use of anterior portals is sufficient to treat most lesions in the knee, such as:

- Meniscal lesions
- Patellofemoral disorders
- Osteochondral lesions
- Cruciate 'ligament' pathology
- Inflammatory or tumoral pathology of the synovium
- Intra-articular loose bodies

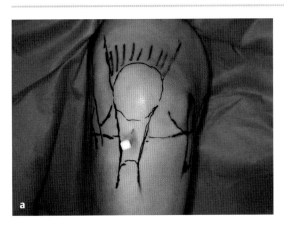
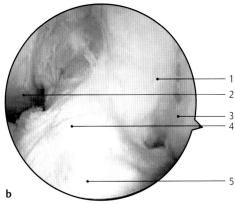

Fig. 5.6   (a) The central transpatellar ligament portal is located 1 cm distal to the inferior pole of the patella at the midline of the patellar ligament. This portal is useful during posterior cruciate ligament reconstruction and as an extra working portal during total meniscectomies or tibial eminence avulsion fracture fixation. **(b)** Arthroscopic view of right knee with the arthroscope through the central transpatellar ligament portal.

1 Femoral origin of the posterior cruciate ligament, 2 Lateral femoral condyle, 3 Medial femoral condyle, 4 Anterior cruciate ligament, 5 Tibial insertion of the anterior cruciate ligament

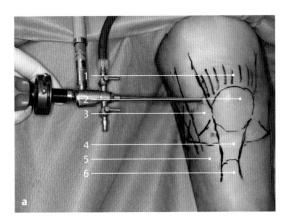
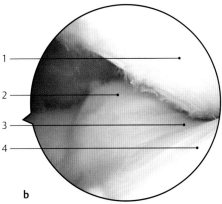

Fig. 5.7   (a) View of right knee in extension with the arthroscope in the superolateral portal and the lens looking distally. **(b)** Arthroscopic view of right knee in extension from the superolateral portal. Note that in this case the arthroscope provides a proximal view and allows further evaluation of the patellofemoral joint and suprapatellar recess.

1 Quadriceps muscle tendon, 2 Patella, 3 Lateral femoral condyle, 4 Patellar ligament, 5 Lateral tibial condyle, 6 Tibial tuberosity, 7 Lateral articular facet of patella, 8 Medial femoral condyle, 9 Intercondylar fossa (trochlea), 10 Lateral femoral condyle

131

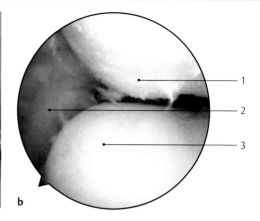

Fig. 5.8 **(a)** Right knee in extension as the arthroscope enters the knee through the superomedial portal, as the lens looks distal. **(b)** Arthroscopic view of right knee and the patellofemoral joint through the superomedial portal.

1 Quadriceps muscle tendon, 2 Patella, 3 Medial femoral condyle, 4 Medial tibial condyle, 5 Patellar ligament, 6 Tibial tuberosity, 7 Medial articular facet of patella, 8 Medial patellar retinaculum, 9 Medial femoral condyle

5.4.1 Anterolateral Portal

The suggested sequence for a diagnostic arthroscopy of the knee via the anterolateral portal is shown in the **Figs. 5.9–5.16**.

1. Introduction of the arthroscope through the anterolateral portal (**Fig. 5.9**)
2. Evaluation of the patellofemoral joint (**Fig. 5.9**)
3. Evaluation of the lateral recess and the popliteus muscle tendon (**Fig. 5.10**)
4. Evaluation of the medial recess (**Fig. 5.11**)
5. Evaluation of the medial femorotibial compartment (**Fig. 5.12**)
6. Location of the anteromedial portal (**Figs. 5.13** and **5.14**)
7. Evaluation of the intercondylar fossa and cruciate ligaments (**Fig. 5.15**)
8. Evaluation of the lateral femorotibial compartment (**Fig. 5.16**)

Once these steps are complete, the surgeon can proceed with the specific procedure, change the orientation of the lens, or move the arthroscope from one portal to another.

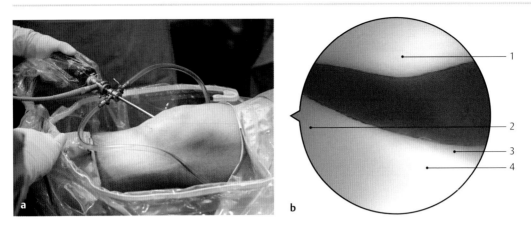

Fig. 5.9 **(a)** Right knee in extension for evaluation of the patellofemoral joint; the arthroscope is in the anterolateral portal. **(b)** Arthroscopic view.

1 Articular surface of the patella, 2 Lateral femoral condyle, 3 Medial femoral condyle, 4 Intercondylar fossa (trochlea)

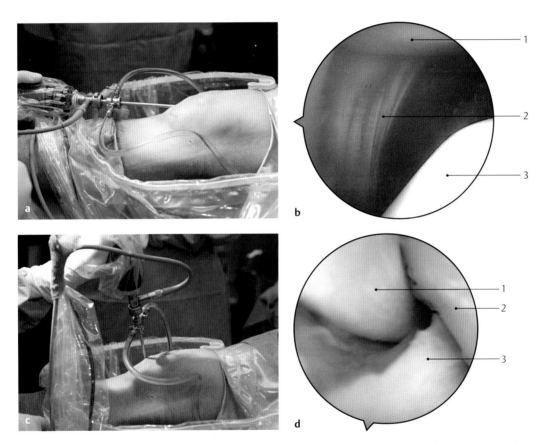

Fig. 5.10 **(a)** Right knee in extension for the evaluation of the lateral recess with the arthroscope through the anterolateral portal, as the lens looks lateral. **(b)** Arthroscopic view. **(c)** View of right knee with the arthroscope in the anterolateral portal, with the lens looking distally for evaluation of the popliteus tendon in the lateral gutter. **(d)** Arthroscopic view.

1 Lateral facet of the patella, 2 Lateral retinaculum, 3 Lateral femoral condyle, 4 Popliteus tendon, 5 Lateral femoral condyle, 6 Lateral meniscus

133

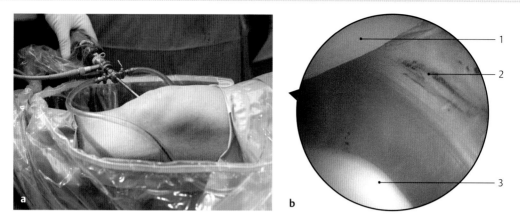

Fig. 5.11 **(a)** Right knee in extension with the arthroscope in the anterolateral portal for evaluation of the medial gutter. **(b)** Arthroscopic view.

1 Patella, 2 Medial retinaculum, 3 Medial femoral condyle

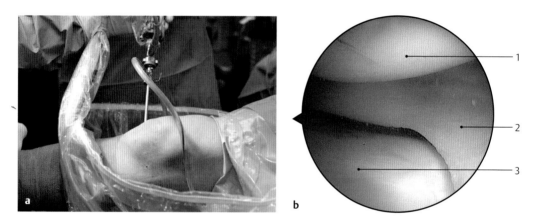

Fig. 5.12 **(a)** Right knee in extension with the arthroscope in the anterolateral portal for evaluation of the medial compartment. **(b)** Arthroscopic view.

1 Medial femoral condyle, 2 Medial meniscus, 3 Medial tibial condyle

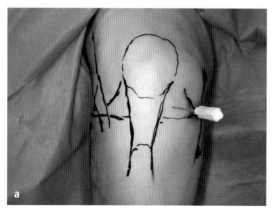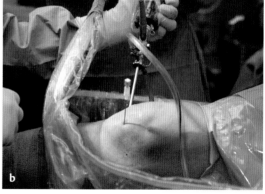

Fig. 5.13 **(a)** Anteromedial portal of the right knee, with the final location marked by a spinal needle and **(b)** checked arthroscopically from the anterolateral portal.

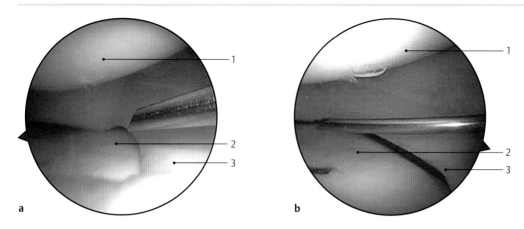

Fig. 5.14 **(a, b)** Arthroscopic view of the right knee from the anterolateral portal; the needle shows the correct location of the anteromedial portal. The rotation of the lens allows a wider field of vision of the medial meniscus and the joint capsule.

1 Medial femoral condyle, 2 Medial tibial condyle, 3 Medial meniscus

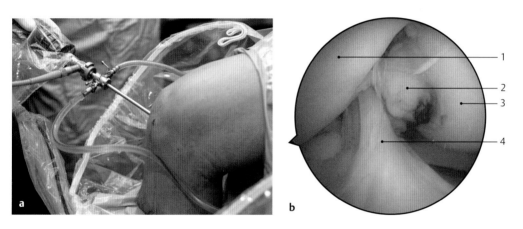

Fig. 5.15 **(a)** Right knee flexed to 90 degrees with the arthroscope in the anterolateral portal for an examination of the intercondylar fossa. The camera is in a vertical position with the lens looking lateral. **(b)** Arthroscopic view.

1 Lateral femoral condyle, 2 Femoral origin of the posterior cruciate ligament, 3 Medial femoral condyle, 4 Anterior cruciate ligament (mucous ligament)

(Continued)

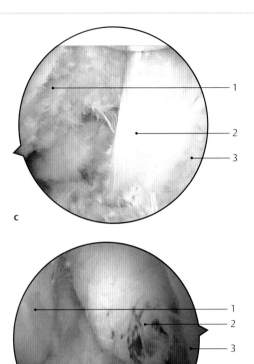

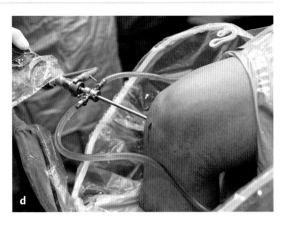

Fig. 5.15 (*continued*) **(c)** Intra-articular view of the right knee (cadaveric) flexed to 90 degrees with the arthroscope in the anterolateral portal. In this case the anterior cruciate ligament is resected to allow a complete visualization of the medial wall of the lateral femoral condyle and the posterior cruciate ligament.

1 Medial wall of the lateral femoral condyle, 2 Posterior cruciate ligament, 3 Medial femoral condyle

(d) Right knee with the arthroscope in the anterolateral portal and the lens rotated to get a medial view. **(e)** Arthroscopic view.

1. Lateral femoral condyle, 2. Femoral origin of the posterior cruciate ligament, 3. Medial femoral condyle 4. Anterior cruciate ligament

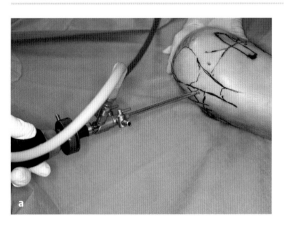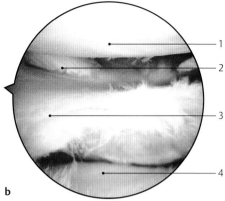

Fig. 5.16 **(a)** Right (cadaveric) knee placed in a figure-of-four position for examination of the lateral femorotibial compartment. The camera should follow the change in the orientation of the articular surface of the knee. **(b)** Arthroscopic view.

1 Lateral femoral condyle, 2 Popliteus muscle tendon, 3 Lateral meniscus (with degenerative changes), 4 Lateral tibial condyle

5.4.2 Anterior Anatomy of the Knee

The infrapatellar branches of the saphenous nerve, as well as the saphenous vein, could be damaged during arthroscopic procedures in the knee (**Fig. 5.17**).

The four main portals (anterolateral, anteromedial, posteromedial, and posterolateral) are marked by Steinmann pins in **Fig. 5.18** to appreciate their spatial relationship.

The anatomical structures—osteoarticular, tendinous, and ligamentous—are shown in **Figs. 5.19–5.23**.

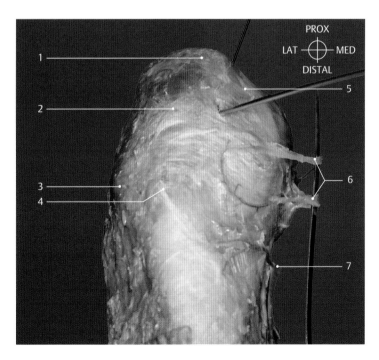

Fig. 5.17 Anterior view of the right knee flexed to 90 degrees shows the subcutaneous structures.

1 Patella
2 Patellar ligament
3 Head of the fibula
4 Tuberosity of the tibia
5 Medial retinaculum of patella
6 Infrapatellar branches of saphenous nerve
7 Great saphenous vein

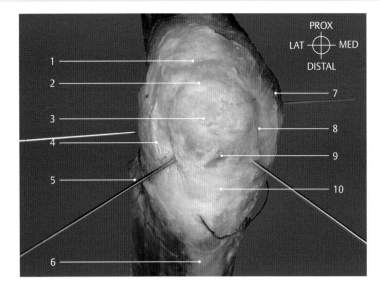

Fig. 5.18 Right knee and the subcutaneous structures related to the anterior portals. The anterior and posterior portals are marked with Steinmann pins.

1 Quadriceps muscle tendon
2 Base of patella
3 Patella
4 Lateral retinaculum of patella
5 Head of the fibula
6 Tibial tuberosity
7 Vastus medialis muscle
8 Medial retinaculum of patella
9 Apex of patella
10 Patellar ligament

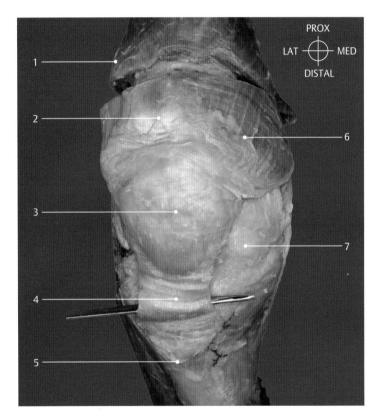

Fig. 5.19 Anterior view of the right knee and its extensor mechanism.

1 Vastus lateralis muscle
2 Rectus femoralis muscle
3 Patella
4 Patellar ligament
5 Tibial tuberosity
6 Vastus medialis muscle
7 Medial retinaculum of patella

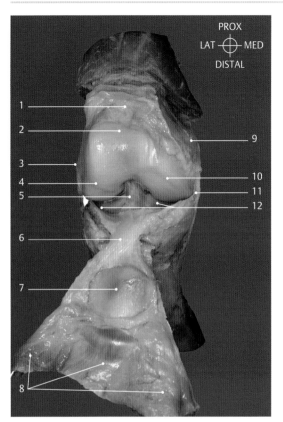

Fig. 5.20 Anterior view of the right knee. The quadriceps muscle tendon is sectioned and taken down to show the anterior intra-articular structures.

1 Suprapatellar bursa
2 Trochlea
3 Lateral collateral ligament
4 Lateral femoral condyle
5 Infrapatellar synovial fold/anterior cruciate ligament
6 Infrapatellar fat pad/patellar ligament
7 Articular surface of patella
8 Quadriceps muscle tendon
9 Adductor tubercle of femur
10 Medial femoral condyle
11 Medial collateral ligament
12 Lateral and medial meniscus

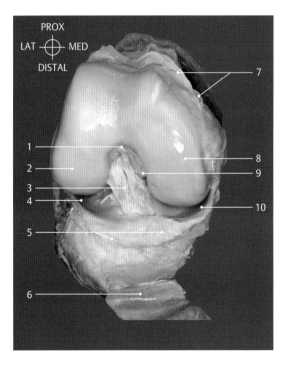

Fig. 5.21 Anterior intra-articular structures of the right knee; the extensor mechanism is cut at the quadriceps tendon and turned down.

1 Intercondylar fossa
2 Lateral femoral condyle
3 Anterior cruciate ligament
4 Lateral meniscus
5 Infrapatellar fat pad
6 Patellar ligament
7 Articular capsule of the knee
8 Medial femoral condyle
9 Posterior cruciate ligament
10 Medial meniscus

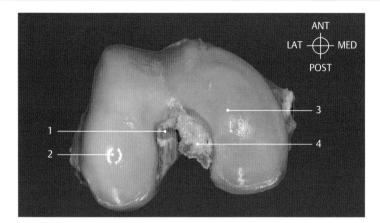

Fig. 5.22   Distal femur of the right knee. Both cruciate ligaments were resected leaving just the insertions.

1 Anterior cruciate ligament
2 Lateral femoral condyle
3 Medial femoral condyle
4 Posterior cruciate ligament

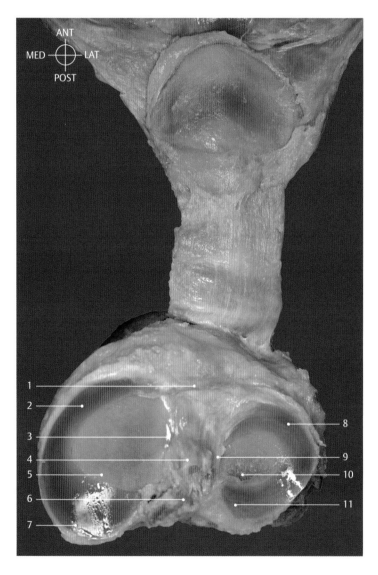

Fig. 5.23   Superior view of the articular surface of the proximal tibia of the right knee.

 1 Transverse ligament of the knee
 2 Anterior horn of the medial meniscus
 3 Medial intercondylar tubercle
 4 Anterior cruciate ligament
 5 Medial tibial condyle
 6 Posterior cruciate ligament
 7 Posterior horn of the medial meniscus
 8 Anterior horn of the lateral meniscus
 9 Lateral intercondylar tubercle
10 Lateral tibial condyle
11 Posterior horn of the lateral meniscus

5.4.3 Lateral Anatomy of the Knee

The lateral anatomical structures of the knee are shown in **Figs. 5.24–5.26**.

5.4.4 Medial Anatomy of the Knee

The anatomical structures of the medial side of the knee are shown in **Figs. 5.27–5.30**.

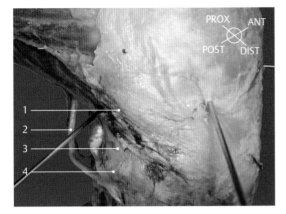

Fig. 5.24 Anterolateral view of the right knee and its subcutaneous structures.

1 Iliotibial tract
2 Biceps femoris muscle tendon
3 Lateral collateral ligament
4 Head of the fibula

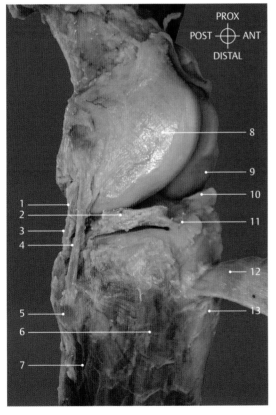

Fig. 5.25 Anterolateral view of the right knee.

1 Popliteus muscle tendon
2 Lateral meniscus
3 Arcuate popliteal ligament
4 Lateral collateral ligament
5 Head of the fibula
6 Tibialis anterior muscle
7 Fibularis longus muscle
8 Lateral femoral condyle
9 Medial femoral condyle
10 Medial meniscus
11 Infrapatellar fat pad
12 Patellar ligament
13 Tibial tuberosity

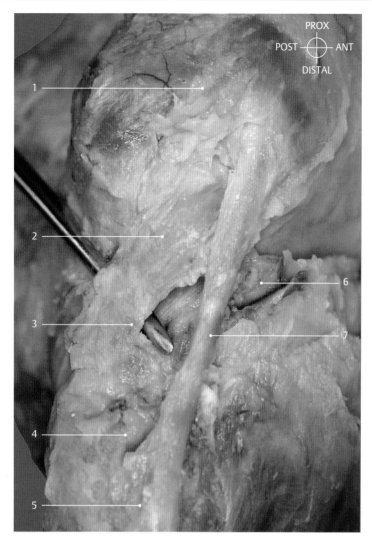

Fig. 5.26 Right knee showing the lateral ligaments and tendons.

1 Lateral femoral condyle
2 Popliteus muscle tendon
3 Arcuate popliteal ligament
4 Biceps femoris muscle tendon (cut)
5 Head of the fibula
6 Lateral meniscus
7 Lateral collateral ligament

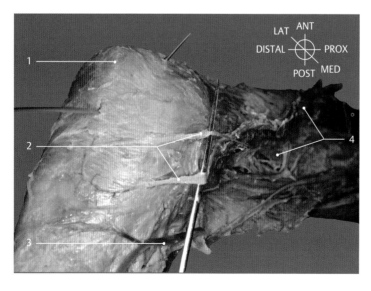

Fig. 5.27 Anteromedial view of the superficial structures of the right knee.

1 Patella
2 Infrapatellar branches of the saphenous nerve
3 Great saphenous vein
4 Vastus medialis muscle (quadriceps muscle)

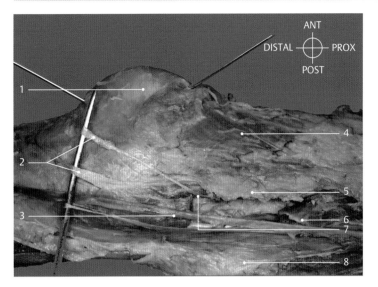

Fig. 5.28 Medial view of the superficial structures of the right knee in extension.

1 Patella
2 Infrapatellar branches of the saphenous nerve
3 Great saphenous vein
4 Vastus medialis muscle (quadriceps muscle)
5 Sartorius muscle
6 Adductor longus muscle
7 Saphenous nerve
8 Adductor magnus muscle

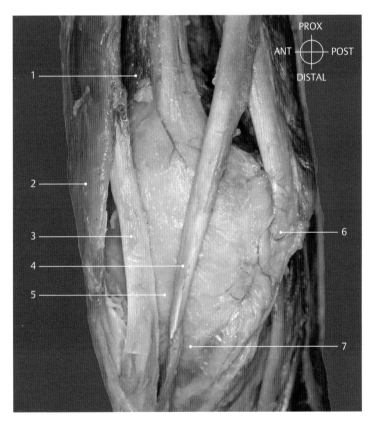

Fig. 5.29 Posteromedial view of the musculotendinous structures of the right knee.

1 Vastus medialis muscle
2 Sartorius muscle
3 Gracilis muscle tendon
4 Semitendinosus muscle tendon
5 Medial femoral condyle
6 Semimembranosus muscle tendon
7 Medial tibial condyle

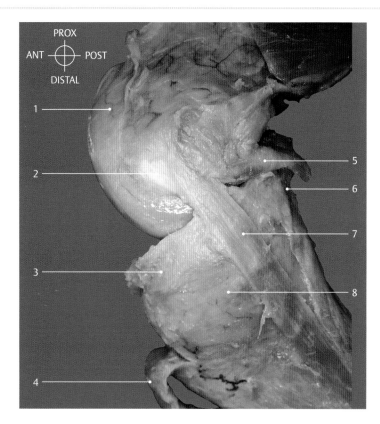

Fig. 5.30 Medial view of the right knee showing the anatomy of the medial collateral ligament from its femoral origin to its tibial attachments.

1 Medial femoral condyle
2 Medial femoral epicondyle
3 Medial meniscus
4 Patellar ligament
5 Medial head of the gastrocnemius muscle
6 Semimembranosus muscle tendon (cut)
7 Medial collateral ligament
8 Medial tibial condyle

5.5 Arthroscopy of the Knee: Posterior

5.5.1 Posterior Portals

The clinical situations in which the knee is treated via the anterior portals are far more frequent than the pathologies approached via posterior portals. However, there are some pathologies mentioned here that can be treated via posterior portals. But, because the posterior anatomy of the knee is complex, these procedures are more difficult and risky.

- Lesions of the posterior cruciate ligament
- Synovium pathologies (villonodular synovitis)
- Lesions of the posterior horn of both menisci
- Intra-articular loose bodies

5.5.2 Posteromedial Portal

The suggested technique and the corresponding arthroscopic views for the posteromedial portal are shown in **Figs. 5.31–5.35**.

1. Identification of the right spot for the posteromedial portal with arthroscopic assistance using the anterolateral portal. The central transpatellar ligament portal is also an option (**Fig. 5.31**).

2. Location of the arthroscope in the posteromedial portal (**Fig. 5.32**).

3. Examination of the posteromedial compartment medial to lateral (**Figs. 5.33–5.35**).

Posteromedial Anatomy of the Knee

To perform a safe arthroscopy of the knee via the posteromedial portal one must know the anatomy well. The main superficial neurovascular structures and a dissection that goes deeper to the capsule are shown in **Figs. 5.36–5.38**; the posteromedial capsule is opened to get an intraarticular view.

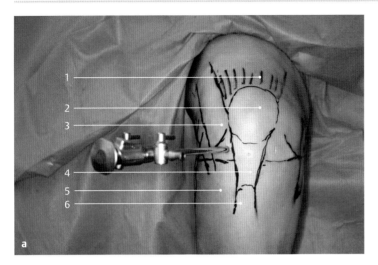

Fig. 5.31 Right (cadaveric) knee with the arthroscope in the anterolateral portal as the first step for a posteromedial arthroscopy of the knee. The arthroscope is advanced posteromedially through the intercondylar fossa. The right spot for the posteromedial portal is found by transillumination of the skin and direct arthroscopic control.

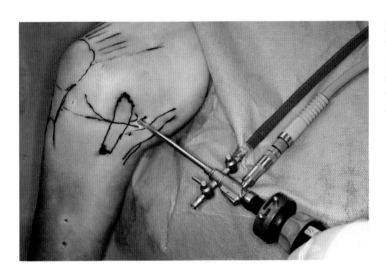

Fig. 5.32 The initial position of the arthroscope in the posteromedial portal in a right (cadaveric) knee. The knee is flexed to 90 degrees with the camera in the vertical position and the lens rotated for an anterior view.

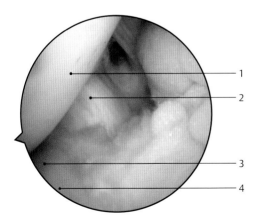

Fig. 5.33 Arthroscopic view through the posteromedial portal in right (cadaveric) knee following the technique shown in **Fig. 5.32**.

1 Medial femoral condyle
2 Posterior cruciate ligament
3 Medial meniscus
4 Medial tibial condyle

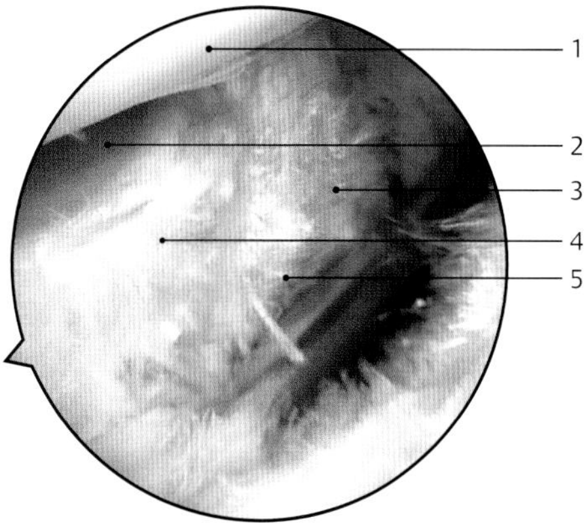

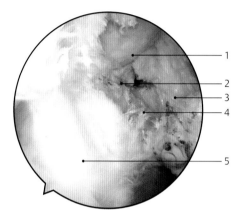

Fig. 5.34 Arthroscopic view of right (cadaveric) knee through the posteromedial portal; the synovium is resected.

1 Medial femoral condyle
2 Posterior horn of the medial meniscus
3 Posterior cruciate ligament
4 Medial tibial condyle
5 Tibial origin of the posterior cruciate ligament

Fig. 5.35 Arthroscopic view of right (cadaveric) knee from the posteromedial portal. The posterior synovium is resected and the arthroscope is advanced lateral.

1 Lateral femoral condyle
2 Lateral meniscus
3 Popliteus muscle tendon
4 Lateral tibial condyle
5 Posterior cruciate ligament

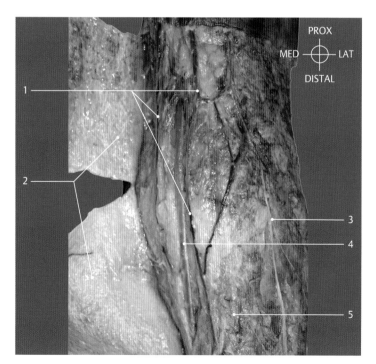

Fig. 5.36 Posterior view of right knee to show the main subcutaneous structures.

1 Genicular veins
2 Skin
3 Terminal branches of posterior femoral cutaneous nerve
4 Great saphenous vein
5 Crural fascia

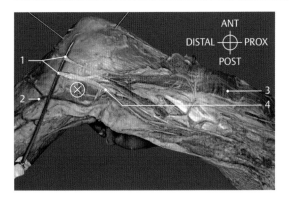

Fig. 5.37   Subcutaneous neurovascular structures of the medial side of the right knee.

1   Infrapatellar branches of saphenous nerve
2   Great saphenous vein
3   Adductor magnus muscle (cut and mobilized)
4   Saphenous nerve
Ⓧ Posteromedial portal

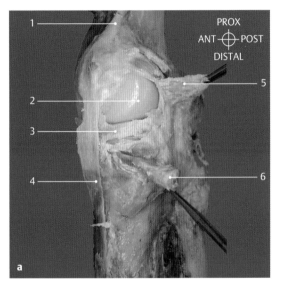

Fig. 5.38   **(a, b)** Posteromedial views of right knee dissected to the posterior capsule and then opened to show the posterior working space.

1   Adductor magnus muscle tendon
2   Medial femoral condyle
3   Medial meniscus
4   Medial collateral ligament
5   Articular capsule
6   Semimembranosus muscle tendon
7   Posterior articular space of the knee

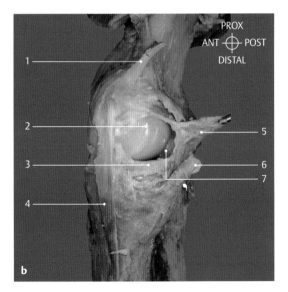

5.5.3 Posterolateral Portal

The suggested sequence for an arthroscopy of the knee via the posterolateral portal is as follows:

1. The location of the posterolateral portal can be found under direct arthroscopic control and transillumination of the skin with the knee flexed to 90 degrees. The arthroscope is typically located in the anteromedial portal (occasionally, the anterolateral or central transpatellar ligament portals are used). The arthroscope is advanced between the anterior cruciate ligament and the lateral femoral condyle (**Figs. 5.39–5.41**).

2. The first anatomical intra-articular landmark in the posterolateral compartment is the lateral femoral condyle; from this point the arthroscope is moved and the lens rotated to identify the lateral meniscus, the popliteus tendon, and the lateral tibial condyle (**Fig. 5.42**).

3. The posteromedial compartment can also be viewed from the posterolateral portal to examine the medial tibial condyle, the medial femoral condyle, and the posterior cruciate ligament (**Fig. 5.43**).

4. Viewing the posterior cruciate ligament at its tibial insertion is also possible from the posterolateral portal (**Fig. 5.43**).

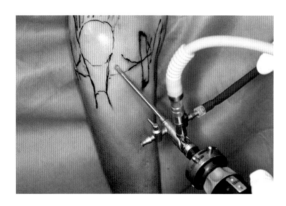

Fig. 5.39   Right (cadaveric) knee with the arthroscope in the anteromedial portal advanced through the intercondylar fossa to locate the posterolateral portal under direct arthroscopic control.

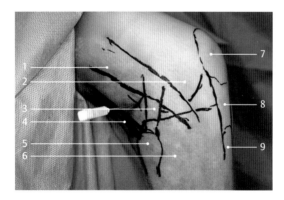

Fig. 5.40   Lateral view of right (cadaveric) knee. The location of the posterolateral portal is marked with a spinal needle and the anatomical landmarks are shown.

1 Iliotibial tract
2 Lateral femoral condyle
3 Lateral collateral ligament
4 Biceps femoris muscle tendon
5 Fibular head
6 Lateral tibial condyle
7 Patella
8 Patellar ligament
9 Tibial tuberosity

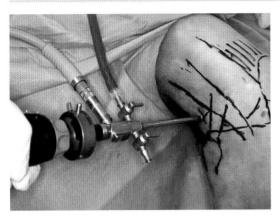

Fig. 5.41 Right (cadaveric) knee with the arthroscope located in the posterolateral portal. The camera is in the vertical position with the lens looking anterior. This setting allows a view of the posterior structures in the knee, as shown in **Fig. 5.42**.

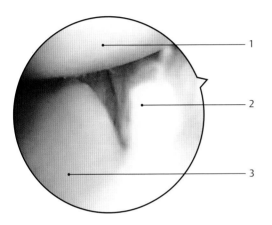

Fig. 5.42 Arthroscopic view of right (cadaveric) knee via the posterolateral portal.

1 Lateral femoral condyle
2 Popliteus muscle tendon
3 Posterior horn of the lateral meniscus

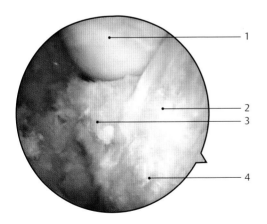

Fig. 5.43 Arthroscopic view of right (cadaveric) knee to evaluate the posteromedial part of the joint via the posterolateral portal.

1 Medial femoral condyle
2 Posterior cruciate ligament
3 Medial tibial condyle
4 Tibial origin of the posterior cruciate ligament

Posterolateral Anatomy of the Knee

The location of the arthroscope in the posterolateral portal is shown in **Fig. 5.44** and the dissection of the lateral and posterolateral anatomy of the knee is presented in **Figs. 5.45–5.48**.

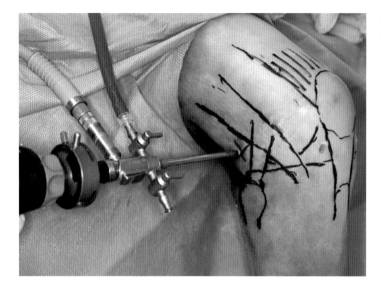

Fig. 5.44   Right (cadaveric) knee with the arthroscope in the posterolateral portal.

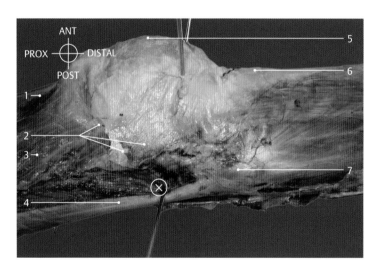

Fig. 5.45   Lateral view of the right knee in extension. The location of the posterolateral portal is marked. The iliotibial tract was resected. In extension the posterolateral structures are tight, including the biceps femoris tendon. This shows the importance of performing a posterior arthroscopy with the knee flexed.

1 Rectus femoris muscle, 2 Iliotibial tract (cut), 3 Vastus lateralis muscle, 4 Biceps femoris muscle tendon, 5 Patella, 6 Tibial tuberosity, 7 Fibular head, Ⓧ Posterolateral portal

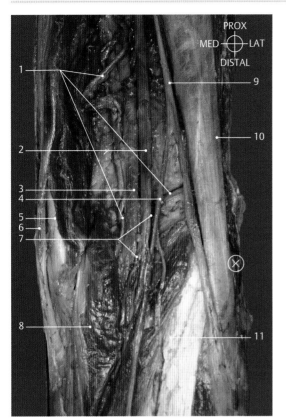

Fig. 5.46   Posterior view of the right knee showing the relation of the posterolateral portal with the neurovascular structures. The biceps femoris tendon is anterior to the common fibular nerve; the posterolateral portal should always be anterior to the tendon.

1   Genicular veins
2   Tibial nerve
3   Popliteal vein
4   Lateral sural cutaneous nerve
5   Semimembranosus muscle tendon
6   Semitendinosus muscle tendon
7   Muscular branches of tibial nerve
8   Medial head of the gastrocnemius muscle
9   Common fibular nerve
10   Biceps femoris muscle tendon
11   Lateral head of the gastrocnemius muscle
(x) Posterolateral portal

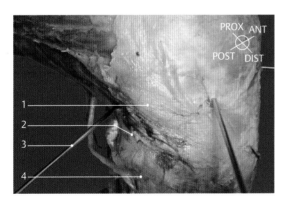

Fig. 5.47   Right knee flexed to 90 degrees; the posterolateral portal is marked with a Steinmann pin. Note there is no tension in the biceps femoris tendon when the knee is flexed.

1   Iliotibial tract
2   Lateral collateral ligament
3   Biceps femoris muscle tendon
4   Fibular head

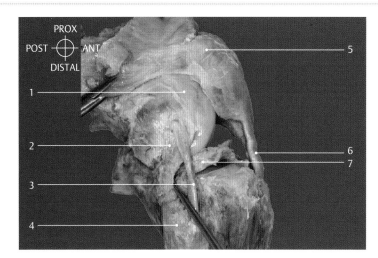

Fig. 5.48 Right knee and its lateral and posterolateral structures.

1 Lateral femoral condyle
2 Popliteus muscle tendon
3 Lateral collateral ligament
4 Fibular head,
5 Patella
6 Patellar ligament
7 Lateral meniscus

5.5.4 Additional Aspects

The posterior anatomy of the knee is complex and a lack of the appropriate anatomical knowledge can lead to serious complications. This is valid for both posterior portals and is detailed in **Figs. 5.49–5.55**.

Axial-sagittal-coronal Views

Please see **Figs. 5.56–5.61** for axial-sagittal-coronal views.

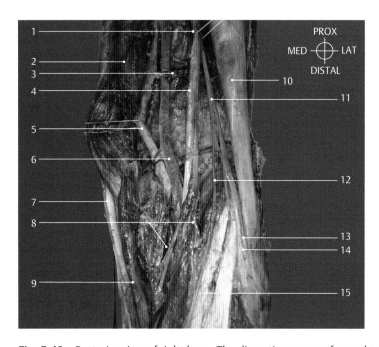

Fig. 5.49 Posterior view of right knee. The dissection was performed to the gastrocnemius muscle layer.

1 Sciatic nerve, 2 Semimembranosus muscle, 3 Lateral superior genicular artery, 4 Tibial nerve, 5 Popliteal artery, 6 Popliteal vein, 7 Semitendinosus muscle tendon, 8 Muscular branches of tibial nerve, 9 Medial head of the gastrocnemius muscle, 10 Biceps femoris muscle tendon, 11 Common fibular nerve, 12 Lateral sural cutaneous nerve, 13 Superficial fibular nerve, 14 Deep fibular nerve, 15 Lateral head of the gastrocnemius muscle

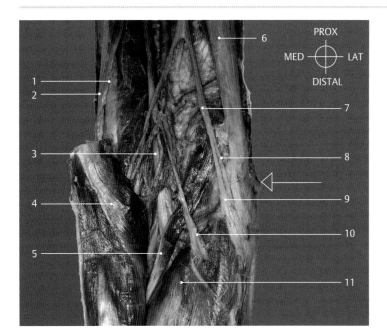

Fig. 5.50   Posterior view of a right knee with the gastrocnemius muscles moved away.

1 Semimembranosus muscle tendon, 2 Semitendinosus muscle tendon, 3 Tibial nerve, 4 Medial head of the gastrocnemius muscle, 5 Plantaris muscle, 6 Biceps femoris muscle tendon, 7 Common fibular nerve, 8 Superficial fibular nerve, 9 Deep fibular nerve, 10 Muscular branches of tibial nerve, 11 Soleus muscle, ← Posterolateral portal

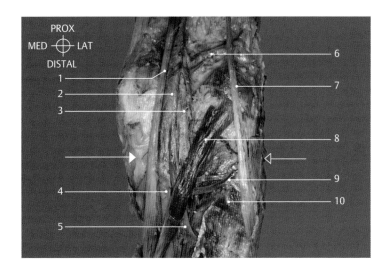

Fig. 5.51   Further posterior dissection of right knee: the muscles were all resected and just the plantaris muscle is still in place.

1 Tibial nerve, 2 Popliteal vein, 3 Popliteal artery, 4 Posterior tibial vein, 5 Anterior tibial vein, 6 Superior lateral genicular vein and artery, 7 Common fibular nerve, 8 Plantaris muscle, 9 Lateral inferior genicular artery and vein, 10 Popliteus muscle, ← Posterolateral portal, ← Posteromedial portal

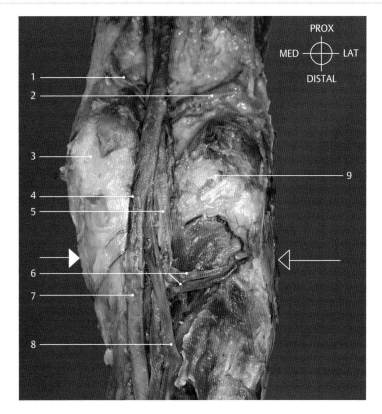

Fig. 5.52 Vascular structures of the posterior knee. Notice the superficial and lateral position of the popliteal vein to the popliteal artery at the distal femur: the vein passes distally to a posterior position and finally to a medial position in relation to the artery.

1 Medial superior genicular vessels
2 Lateral superior genicular vessels
3 Medial femoral condyle
4 Popliteal vein
5 Popliteal artery
6 Lateral inferior genicular vessels
7 Posterior tibial vein
8 Anterior tibial vein
9 Lateral femoral condyle
⇐ Posterolateral portal
← Posteromedial portal

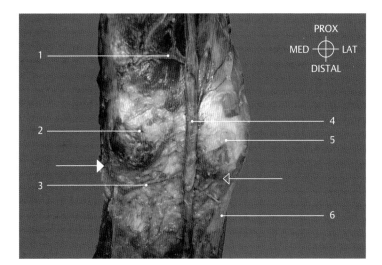

Fig. 5.53 Popliteal artery and genicular branches in the right knee.

1 Medial superior genicular artery
2 Medial femoral condyle
3 Medial inferior genicular artery
4 Popliteal artery
5 Lateral femoral condyle
6 Popliteus muscle tendon
⇐ Posterolateral portal
← Posteromedial portal

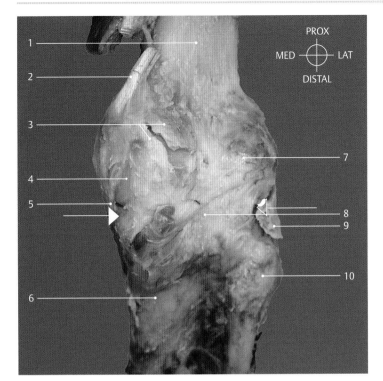

Fig. 5.54 Posterior view of the right knee; the posterior joint capsule layer is shown.

1 Femur
2 Adductor magnus muscle
3 Articular capsule of knee
4 Medial femoral condyle
5 Medial collateral ligament
6 Tibia
7 Lateral femoral condyle
8 Oblique popliteal ligament
9 Arcuate popliteal ligament/ popliteus muscle tendon
10 Fibular head
← Posterolateral portal
← Posteromedial portal

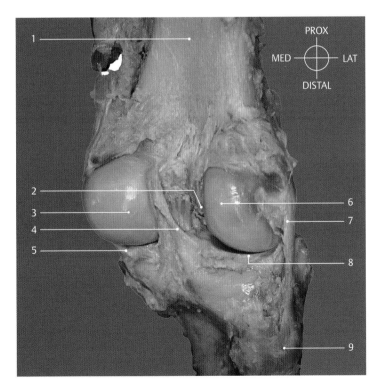

Fig. 5.55 Posterior view of a right knee with the posterior capsule resected.

1 Femur
2 Anterior cruciate ligament (femoral insertion)
3 Medial femoral condyle
4 Posterior meniscofemoral ligament
5 Medial meniscus
6 Lateral femoral condyle
7 Lateral collateral ligament
8 Lateral meniscus
9 Head of the fibula

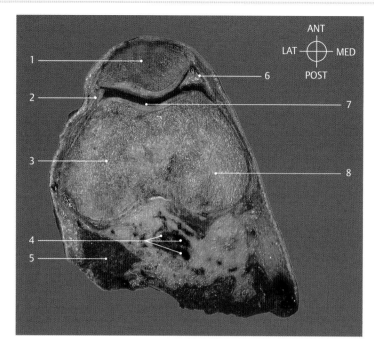

Fig. 5.56 Distal view of an axial cut of the right knee at the level of both femoral condyles and the middle third of the patella.

1 Patella
2 Lateral retinaculum of patella
3 Lateral femoral condyle
4 Popliteal vessels
5 Biceps femoris muscle
6 Medial retinaculum of patella
7 Patellofemoral joint
8 Medial femoral condyle

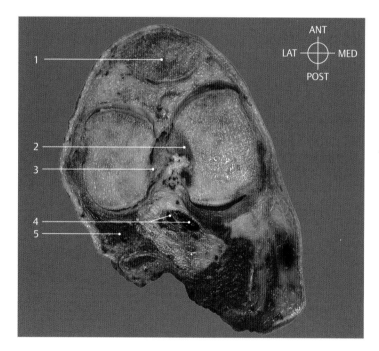

Fig. 5.57 Axial cut of the right knee at the level of the intercondylar fossa—both cruciate ligaments can be identified (inferior view).

1 Patella
2 Posterior cruciate ligament
3 Anterior cruciate ligament
4 Popliteal vessels
5 Biceps femoris muscle

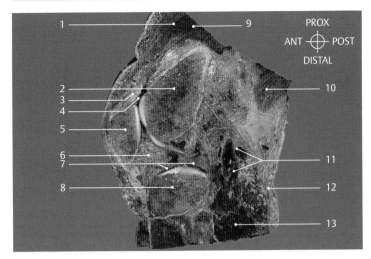

Fig. 5.58 Sagittal cut of the right knee at the lateral tibial condyle.

1 Rectus femoris muscle
2 Lateral femoral condyle
3 Quadriceps muscle tendon
4 Suprapatellar bursa
5 Patella
6 Infrapatellar fat pad
7 Lateral meniscus
8 Lateral tibial condyle
9 Vastus intermedius muscle
10 Biceps femoris muscle
11 Popliteal vessels
12 Crural fascia
13 Lateral gastrocnemius muscle

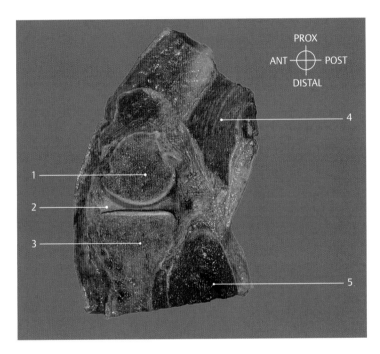

Fig. 5.59 Sagittal cut of the right knee at the level of the medial tibial condyle.

1 Medial femoral condyle
2 Medial meniscus
3 Tibia
4 Semimembranosus muscle
5 Medial head of gastrocnemius muscle

157

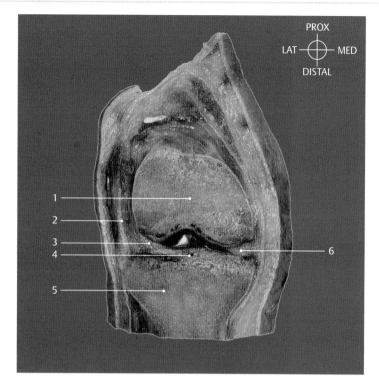

Fig. 5.60 Anterior coronal cut of the right knee.

1 Femur
2 Iliotibial tract
3 Lateral meniscus
4 Lateral intercondylar tubercle
5 Tibia
6 Medial meniscus

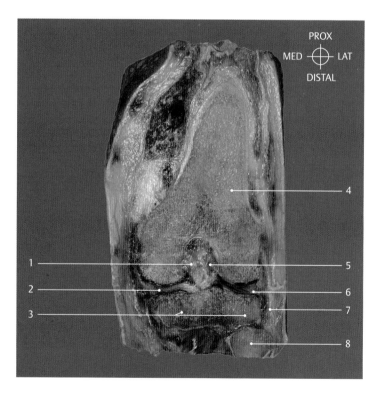

Fig. 5.61 Posterior coronal cut of the right knee.

1 Posterior cruciate ligament
2 Medial meniscus
3 Tibia
4 Femur
5 Anterior cruciate ligament
6 Lateral meniscus
7 Lateral collateral ligament
8 Fibular head

6 Ankle

Cristian Blanco Moreno, Gerardo Muñoz Muraro, Eduardo Vega Pizarro, and Juan Pablo Quinteros Pomar

6.1 Introduction

Ankle arthroscopy allows a direct examination of the intra-articular anatomy of the ankle without the need for an open arthrotomy or malleolar osteotomies; therefore, reducing morbidity and providing faster postoperative recovery. An accurate knowledge of the anatomy of this joint allows the performance of a safe arthroscopy and avoids complications. This chapter reviews the anterior and posterior approaches and their related portals and anatomy.

6.2 Anterior Ankle

The most frequently used portals are the anterolateral and anteromedial. The correct location of these portals avoids damage to the related structures during instrumentation, and depends mostly on the superficial anatomy of the anterior ankle. Other portals are less popular because of the risk of neurovascular complications. This is the case with the anterocentral portal, which is only briefly mentioned in this chapter.

6.2.1 Anatomical Landmarks of the Anterior Ankle

Knowledge of the superficial anatomy of the ankle is crucial for the safe location of the anterior portals. The neurovascular and tendinous structures are most at risk of injury during the procedure. The key landmarks are shown in **Fig. 6.1**.

6.2.2 Therapeutic Indications for Ankle Arthroscopy via Anterior Portals

The therapeutic indications for ankle arthroscopy via anterior portals are:

- Removal of loose bodies
- Synovial biopsy and synovectomy
- Chondral or osteochondral lesions of the talus and tibial plafond
- Excision of soft tissue impinging lesions
- Excision of osteophytes at the tibia and talus
- Intra-articular evaluation of clinically unstable ankles
- Fractures of the tibial plafond and ankle
- Arthroscopically assisted arthrodesis of the ankle
- Septic arthritis of the ankle

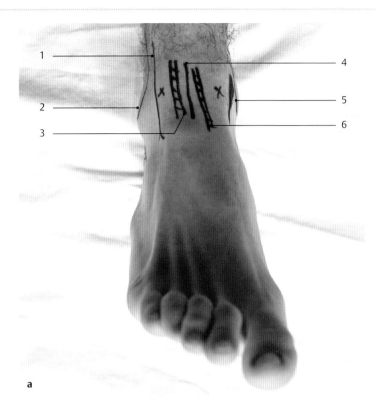

Fig. 6.1 **(a)** Anterior, **(b)** anterolateral, and **(c)** antero medial views of the right ankle. **(c)** Anteromedial view of the right ankle.

1 Superficial fibular nerve
2 Lateral malleolus
3 Extensor digitorum longus tendon
4 Dorsalis pedis artery
5 Medial malleolus
6 Tibialis anterior tendon
7 Great saphenous vein and saphenous nerve
"X" Portals (lateral and medial)

a

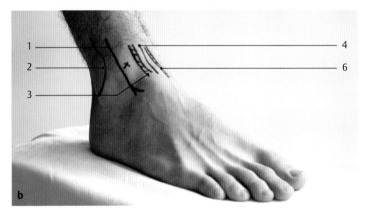

b

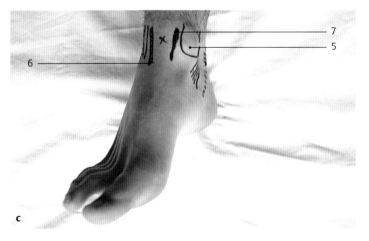

c

6.2.3 Patient Positioning

For an anterior arthroscopy of the ankle the patient is placed supine and a tourniquet is used in most cases. Although different options exist, the authors recommend a soft ankle joint distractor held by a metal bar applied to the lateral support of the surgical table as shown in **Fig. 6.2**. The use of an ankle mechanical distractor is optional but seldom needed. It increases the joint space and makes the procedure easier; however, it has some complications and contraindications (open epiphysis). Some intra-articular views shown in this chapter were taken with the help of an ankle distractor.

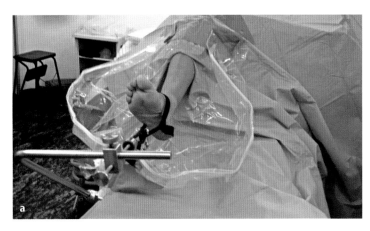

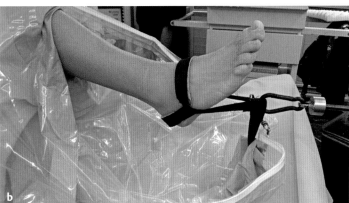

Fig. 6.2 **(a)** Position of the patient for an ankle arthroscopy; a soft tissue harness is used and **(b)** traction is held with the help of a lateral metal bar.

6.2.4 Anterior Portals

Anterolateral Portal

This portal is located at the level of the tibiotalar joint—lateral to the fibularis (peroneus) tertius muscle tendon and extensor digitorum longus muscle tendon (**Fig. 6.3a**).

Anteromedial Portal

This portal is located at the level of the tibiotalar joint, just medial to the tibialis anterior muscle tendon (**Fig. 6.3b**).

Anterocentral Portal

This portal is located at the level of the tibiotalar joint between the extensor hallucis longus tendon and the extensor digitorum longus tendon (**Fig. 6.4**).

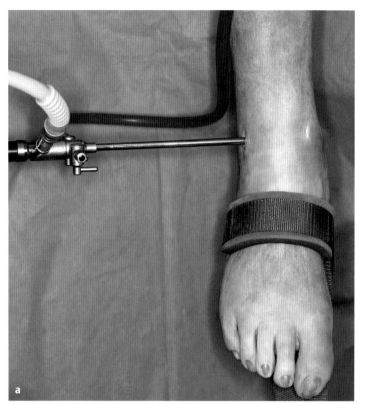

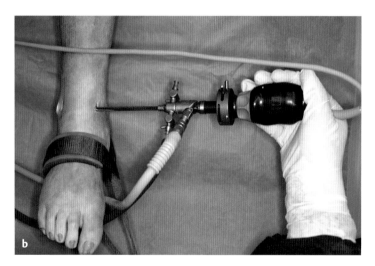

Fig. 6.3 **(a)** Anterior view of a right (cadaveric) ankle with the arthroscope in the anterolateral portal and **(b)** in the anteromedial portal. Regarding the level of the tibiotalar joint, a higher portal makes the exploration of the tibiotalar joint more difficult but facilitates a direct frontal view of the articular surface of the talus. On the other hand, a lower portal makes a direct frontal view of the talus more difficult, but facilitates a direct view of the distal articular surface of the tibia and access to the talar neck.

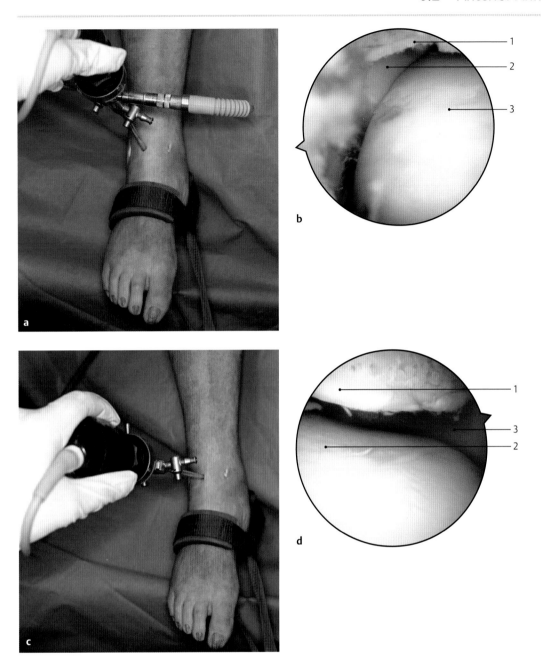

Fig. 6.4 **(a)** Right (cadaveric) ankle with the arthroscope in the anterocentral portal, as the lens looks lateral. **(b)** Arthroscopic view. **(c)** Right (cadaveric) ankle with the arthroscope in the anterocentral portal, as the lens looks medial. **(d)** Arthroscopic view.

1 Distal tibia, 2 Talus, 3 Medial malleolus

6.2.5 Anterior Anatomy of the Ankle and Structures at Risk

The anatomical structures at risk depend on the specific portal to be analyzed. The anatomical dissections in **Figs. 6.5–6.9** help to show the relation of the portals and the neurovascular and tendinous structures at risk.

Anterolateral Portal

For this portal the structures at risk are the superficial fibular nerve and its intermediate dorsal cutaneous branch and the extensor digitorum longus tendon (**Figs. 6.5** and **6.6**).

Anterocentral Portal

For this portal the structures at risk are the medial dorsal cutaneous branch of the superficial fibular nerve at the subcutaneous layer, the tibialis anterior artery at the tendinous layer, and the deep fibular nerve at the subtendinous layer (**Fig. 6.7**).

Anteromedial Portal

For this portal the structures at risk are the tibialis anterior tendon and the great saphenous vein (**Figs. 6.8** and **6.9**).

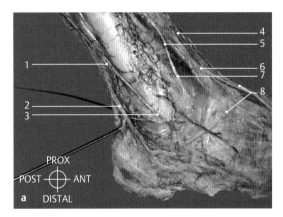

Fig. 6.5   (a) Anterolateral view of a right ankle and the subcutaneous structures, especially the cutaneous branches of the superficial fibular nerve.

1   Sural nerve
2   Lesser saphenous vein
3   Lateral dorsal cutaneous nerve
4   Great saphenous vein
5   Superficial fibular nerve
6   Medial dorsal cutaneous nerve
7   Intermediate dorsal cutaneous nerve
8   Dorsal digital nerves of foot

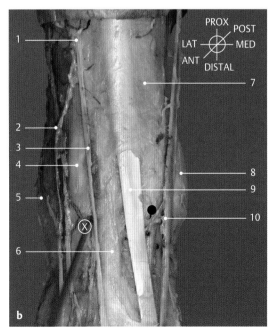

(b) Anterior view of a right ankle and its subcutaneous structures. A Steinmann rod is located at the muscular interval between the extensor digitorum longus and the extensor hallucis longus.

1   Superficial fibular nerve
2   Intermediate dorsal cutaneous nerve
3   Medial dorsal cutaneous nerve
4   Extensor digitorum longus muscle/tendon
5   Lateral malleolus
6   Extensor hallucis longus muscle/tendon
7   Deep fascia
8   Medial malleolus
9   Tibialis anterior muscle/tendon
10   Great saphenous vein
ⓧ Anterolateral portal
●   Anteromedial portal

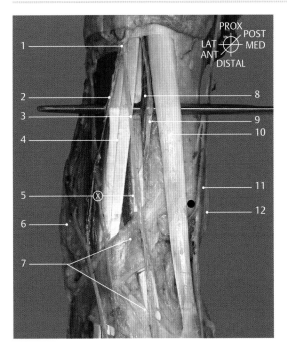

Fig. 6.6 Anterior view of a right ankle showing the tendinous structures and the related neurovascular structures.

1 Superficial fibular nerve
2 Intermediate dorsal cutaneous nerve
3 Medial dorsal cutaneous nerve
4 Extensor digitorum longus muscle/tendon
5 Extensor hallucis longus muscle/tendon
6 Lateral malleolus
7 Extensor retinaculum
8 Anterior tibial artery
9 Deep fibular nerve
10 Tibialis anterior muscle/tendon
11 Great saphenous vein
12 Medial malleolus
(x) Anterolateral portal
● Anteromedial portal

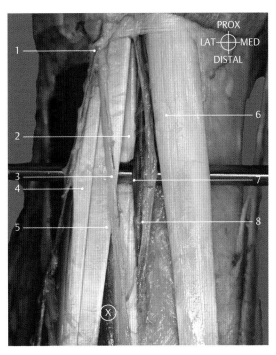

Fig. 6.7 Anterior view of a right ankle with a close-up view of the central neurovascular structures of the ankle joint.

1 Superficial fibular nerve
2 Extensor hallucis longus muscle/tendon
3 Medial dorsal cutaneous nerve
4 Intermediate dorsal cutaneous nerve
5 Extensor digitorum longus muscle/tendon
6 Tibialis anterior muscle/
    tendon
7 Tibialis anterior artery
8 Deep fibular nerve
(x) Anterocentral portal

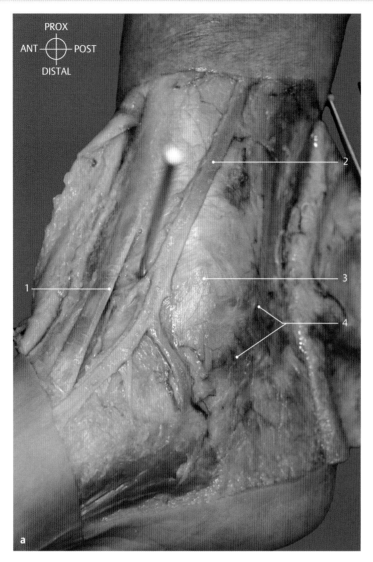

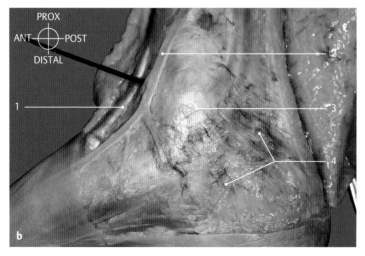

Fig. 6.8   (a, b) Anteromedial and medial views of a right ankle showing the location of the anteromedial portal in relation to the tibialis anterior tendon and the great saphenous vein. The anteromedial portal is marked with a Steinmann rod.

1   Tibialis anterior muscle tendon
2   Great saphenous vein
3   Medial malleolus
4   Flexor retinaculum

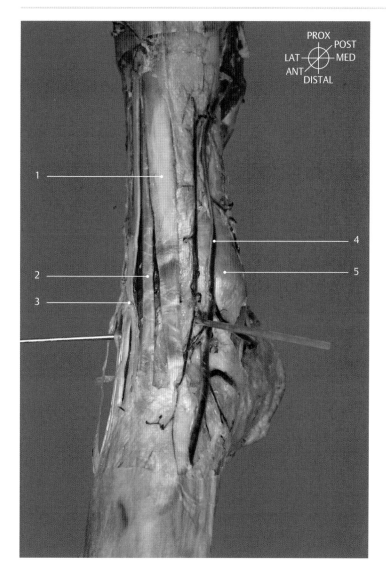

Fig. 6.9   Anteromedial and medial views of a right ankle showing the location of the anteromedial portal in relation to the tibialis anterior tendon and the great saphenous vein. The anteromedial portal is marked with a Steinmann rod.

1 Tibialis anterior muscle/tendon
2 Extensor hallucis longus tendon
3 Extensor digitorum longus muscle/tendon
4 Great saphenous vein
5 Medial malleolus

167

Osteoligamentous Structures

The osteoarticular structures and ligaments of the ankle (anterior, lateral, and medial) can be examined and treated arthroscopically using anterior portals (**Fig. 6.10**).

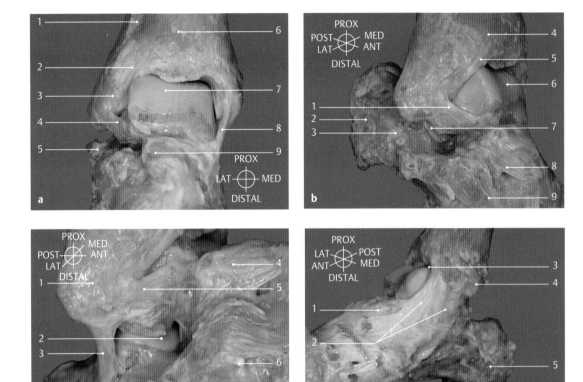

Fig. 6.10   **(a)** Anterior view of a right ankle.

1 Interosseous membrane, 2 Anterior tibiofibular ligament, 3 Fibula, 4 Anterior talofibular ligament, 5 Calcaneofibular ligament (cut), 6 Tibia, 7 Talus, 8 Deltoid ligament, 9 Talonavicular joint

(b) Anterolateral view of a right ankle.

1 Anterior talofibular ligament, 2 Calcaneus, 3 Calcaneofibular ligament cut, 4 Tibia, 5 Anterior tibiofibular ligament, 6 Trochlea of the talus, 7 Subtalar joint, 8 Talonavicular ligament, 9 Calcaneocuboid ligament

(c) Lateral view of a right ankle showing the lateral ligaments. Notice the position of the anterior talofibular ligament when the ankle is in dorsiflexion.

1 Lateral malleolus, 2 Subtalar Joint, 3 Calcaneofibular ligament, 4 Talonavicular ligament, 5 Anterior talofibular ligament, 6 Calcaneocuboid ligament

(d) Anteromedial view of a right ankle.

1 Talonavicular ligament, 2 Deltoid ligament, 3 Talocrural Joint, 4 Medial malleolus, 5 Calcaneus

6.2.6 Arthroscopic Examination of the Ankle via the Anterolateral Portal

Figs. 6.11–6.16 show the arthroscopic approach of the ankle starting with the anterolateral portal; however, some surgeons prefer the anteromedial portal as the starting portal.

After positioning the patient and completing routine sterile preparation and draping, the anatomical landmarks are established (as explained previously). The sites for the portals are confirmed by introducing saline solution through a no. 18 needle into the joint. The incision should be skin deep, with blunt dissection to reach the capsule and avoid injury to the neurovascular structures. **Figs. 6.11–6.16** show the arthroscopic

sequence suggested when using the anterolateral portal first. The decision to perform invasive (osseous) distraction is generally made at the time of the surgery and depends on both the laxity of the ankle joint and the location of the lesion.

1. Superficial anatomical landmarks (**Fig. 6.11**)
2. Anterolateral portal location (**Fig. 6.12**)
3. Arthroscopic view of the anteromedial corner and medial recess (**Fig. 6.13**)
4. Arthroscopic view of the posterior ankle from the anterolateral portal (**Fig. 6.14**)
5. Arthroscopic view of the lateral recess, anterolateral corner, and anterior talofibular ligament (**Fig. 6.15**)
6. Arthroscopic view of the talar neck (**Fig. 6.16**)

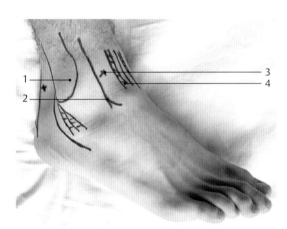

Fig. 6.11   External anatomical landmarks.

1 Lateral malleolus
2 Intermediate dorsal cutaneous branch of the superficial fibular nerve
3 Anterolateral portal
4 Extensor digitorum longus muscle tendon

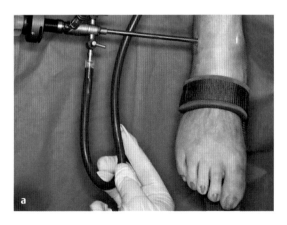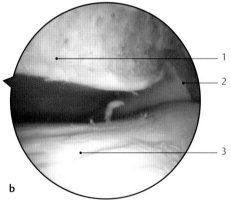

Fig. 6.12   **(a)** Right (cadaveric) ankle with the arthroscope in the anterolateral portal.
(b) Arthroscopic view.

1 Distal tibia, 2 Medial malleolus, 3 Talus

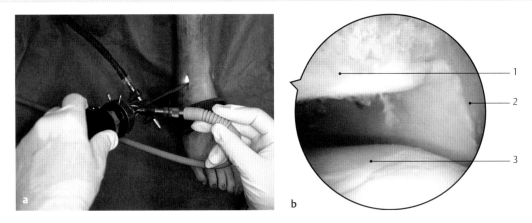

Fig. 6.13   **(a)** Right (cadaveric) ankle with the arthroscope through the anterolateral portal. The position of the arthroscope and the lens allows a view of the medial recess. **(b)** Arthroscopic view.

1 Distal tibia, 2 Medial malleolus, 3 Talus

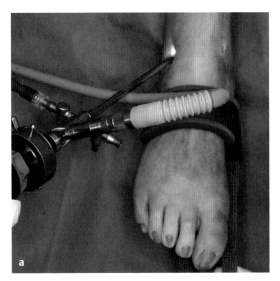

Fig. 6.14   **(a)** Right (cadaveric) ankle with the arthroscope in the anterolateral portal and the lens looking lateral to evaluate the posterocentral and posterolateral tibiotalar joint (under distraction). **(b)** Arthroscopic posterior central view. **(c)** Arthroscopic posterolateral view.

1 Articular surface of the tibia
2 Posterior joint capsule
3 Articular surface of the talus

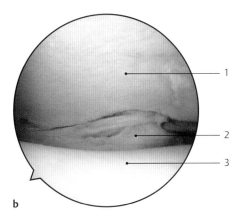

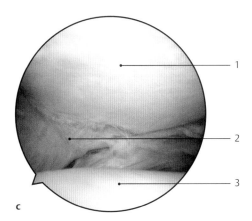

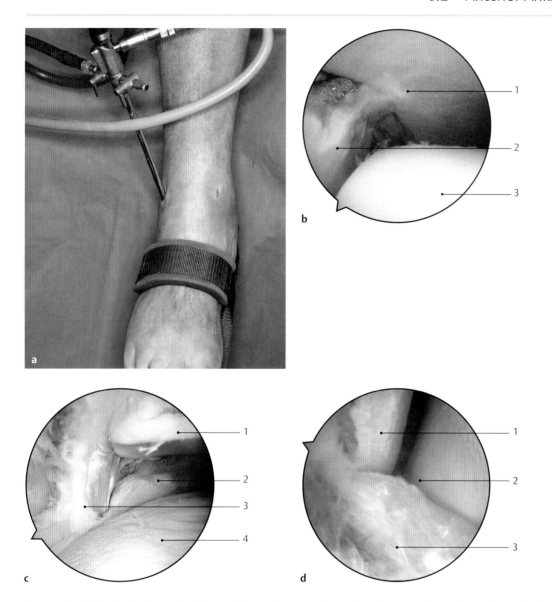

Fig. 6.15 **(a)** Right (cadaveric) ankle with the arthroscope located in the anterolateral portal and the lens rotated to see the lateral recess, anterolateral corner, and anterior talofibular ligament (under distraction). **(b)** Arthroscopic view, lateral gutter.

1 Articular surface of the tibia, 2 Distal fibula, 3 Articular surface of the talus

(c) Arthroscopic view, anterolateral corner.

1 Distal tibia, 2 Distal fibula (part of the talofibular joint), 3 Anterior tibiofibular ligament, 4 Talus

(d) Arthroscopic view, anterior talofibular ligament.

1 Distal fibula, 2 Lateral talus (part of the talofibular joint), 3 Anterior talofibular ligament

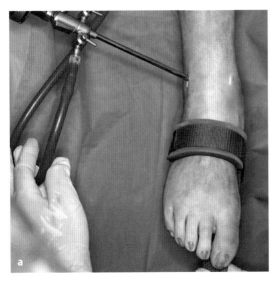
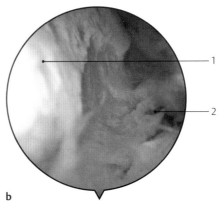

Fig. 6.16 **(a)** Right (cadaveric) ankle with the arthroscope in the anterolateral portal and the lens rotated to look at the talar neck. **(b)** Arthroscopic view, talar neck.

1 Articular surface of the talus, 2 Talar neck

6.2.7 Arthroscopy of the Ankle Using the Anteromedial Portal

A brief sequence of this approach is shown in **Figs. 6.17**–**6.20**. The use of invasive distraction is optional.

1. Establish the anteromedial portal and evaluate the talus and the anterolateral corner (**Fig. 6.17**)

2. Check the anterolateral portal location (**Fig. 6.18**)

3. Evaluate the anteromedial corner, talar dome, and distal tibia (**Fig. 6.19**)

4. View of the talar neck (**Fig. 6.20**)

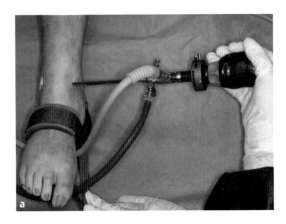
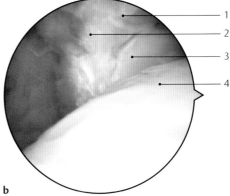

Fig. 6.17 **(a)** A right (cadaveric) ankle with the arthroscope in the anteromedial portal, the lens looks medially but shows the anterolateral corner and talus. **(b)** Arthroscopic view.
1 Tibia, 2 Anterior tibiofibular ligament, 3 Fibula (part of the talofibular joint), 4 Talus

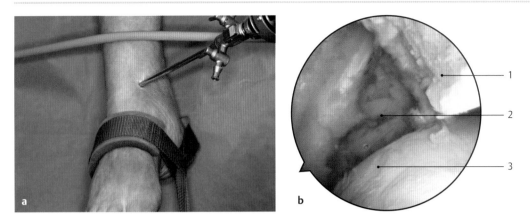

Fig. 6.18   (a) Right (cadaveric) ankle with the arthroscope in the anteromedial portal and the lens rotated to look anteriorly, which is useful to locate the anterolateral portal. **(b)** Arthroscopic view.

1 Anterior border of the distal tibia, 2 Location of the anterolateral portal, 3 Articular surface of the talus

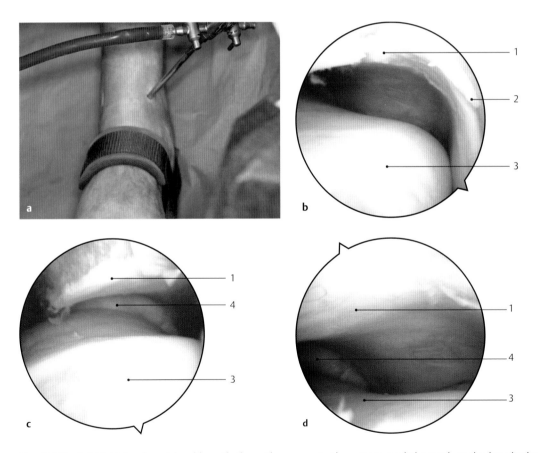

Fig. 6.19   (a) Right (cadaveric) ankle with the arthroscope in the anteromedial portal, as the lens looks at the anteromedial corner. Then the lens is rotated to look distally and later proximally for the following arthroscopic views. **(b)** Arthroscopic view, anteromedial corner.

1 Distal tibia, 2 Medial malleolus, 3 Articular surface of the talus, 4 Fibula

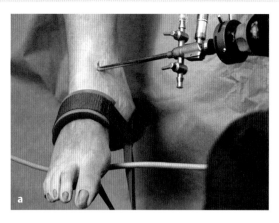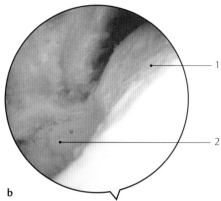

Fig. 6.20 **(a)** Right (cadaveric) ankle with the arthroscope in the anteromedial corner, as the lens looks at the talar neck and part of the articular surface of the talus. **(b)** Arthroscopic view.

1 Articular surface of the talus, 2 Talar neck

6.3 Posterior Ankle

The anatomical landmarks for the posterior portals are less complex than for the anterior portals. However, the technique for installing the portals should be meticulous and the arthroscopic working space has to be carefully respected to prevent injury to important deep neurovascular structures, especially at the medial side. The classic portals are the posterolateral and the posteromedial portals and are discussed here thoroughly.

6.3.1 Anatomical Landmarks of the Posterior Ankle

The superficial anatomical landmarks of the posterior ankle are shown in **Figs. 6.21** and **6.22**.

6.3.2 Therapeutic Indications for Ankle Arthroscopy via Posterior Portals

The following pathologies are treated via posterior arthroscopy of the ankle:

- Common synovitis
- Other synovitis (villonodular, synovial chondromatosis)
- Impingement (osteophytes, os trigonum)
- Posterior soft tissue impingement
- Osteochondral lesions of the talus and subtalar joint (subtalar arthrodesis)
- Septic arthritis

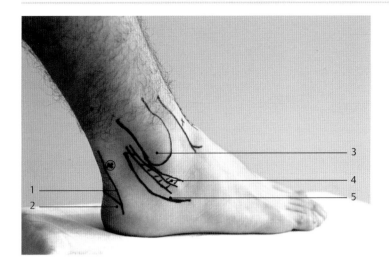

Fig. 6.21   The posterolateral anatomy of the ankle shown from posterior to anterior.

1 Calcaneus tendon
2 Calcaneal tuberosity
3 Lateral malleolus
4 Fibularis tendons
5 Sural nerve and lesser saphenous vein
(X) Posterolateral portal

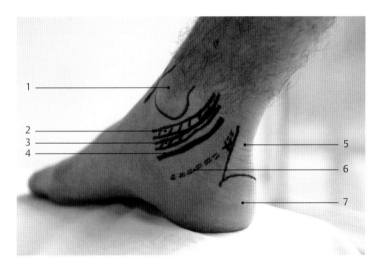

Fig. 6.22   The posteromedial anatomy of the ankle shown from anterior to posterior.

1 Medial malleolus
2 Tibialis posterior muscle tendon
3 Flexor digitorum longus muscle tendon
4 Posterior tibial neurovascular bundle
5 Calcaneus tendon
6 Flexor hallucis longus muscle tendon (discontinuous lines because it is far more deep)
7 Calcaneal tuberosity

6.3.3 Patient Positioning

The setting for a posterior ankle arthroscopy is usually simple. The patient is prone with the foot off the edge of the table and elevated (compare with the opposite limb as shown in **Fig. 6.23**). Distraction (invasive or not) is used as needed. Free dorsiflexion must be possible in this setting.

6.3.4 Posterior Portals

Posterolateral Portal

This portal is established just lateral to the calcaneus tendon, at the level of the posterior articu-

lar line, ~1 cm distal to the anterior articular line and 1 or 1.5 cm proximal to the distal tip of the fibula (**Fig. 6.24**).

Posteromedial portal

This portal is located just medial to the calcaneus tendon at the level of the posterior tibiotalar joint line. This portal should be established with extreme care because of the proximity of the posterior tibial artery, tibial nerve, and tendons (flexor hallucis longus, flexor digitorum longus). For this reason some surgeons prefer the transcalcaneus tendon portal (**Fig. 6.25**).

175

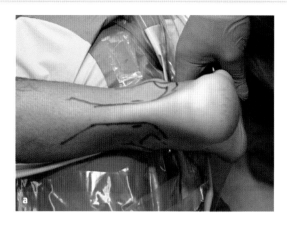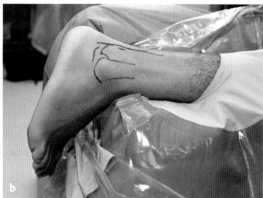

Fig. 6.23 (a, b) Position of the patient for an arthroscopy of the posterior right ankle. Distraction was not used in this case.

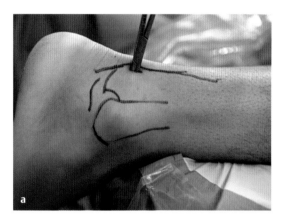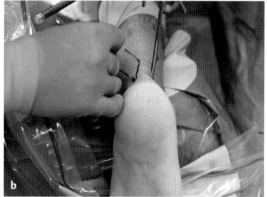

Fig. 6.24 (a, b) Lateral and posterior views of a right ankle showing the position for the posterolateral portal.

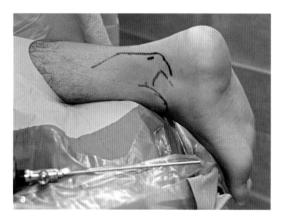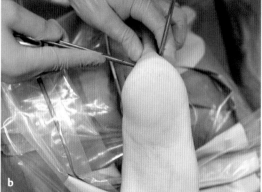

Fig. 6.25 (a, b) Lateral and posterior views of a right ankle showing the position for the posteromedial portal.

6.3.5 Posterior Anatomy of the Ankle and Structures at Risk

The anatomical structures at risk depend on the specific portal that is being used. The anatomical dissections illustrated in **Figs. 6.26–6.28** show the relationship between the portals and the neurovascular and tendinous structures at risk.

Posterolateral Portal

For this portal the structures at risk are the small saphenous vein, the sural nerve (consistently posterior and deeper to the vein), and the calcaneus tendon (**Figs. 6.26** and **6.27**).

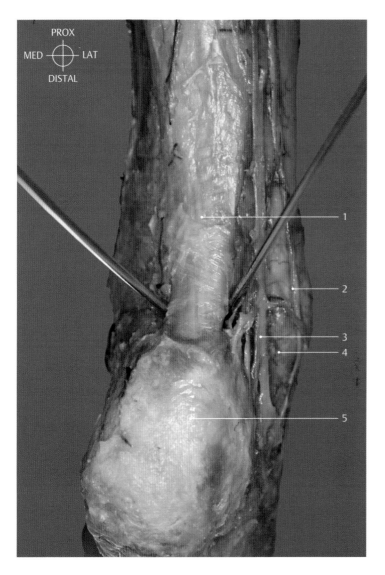

Fig. 6.26 Posterior view of a right ankle with both posterior portals (medial and lateral) marked by Steinmann rods.

1 Calcaneus tendon
2 Sural nerve (lateral dorsal cutaneous branch)
3 Lesser saphenous vein
4 Lateral malleolus
5 Calcaneus

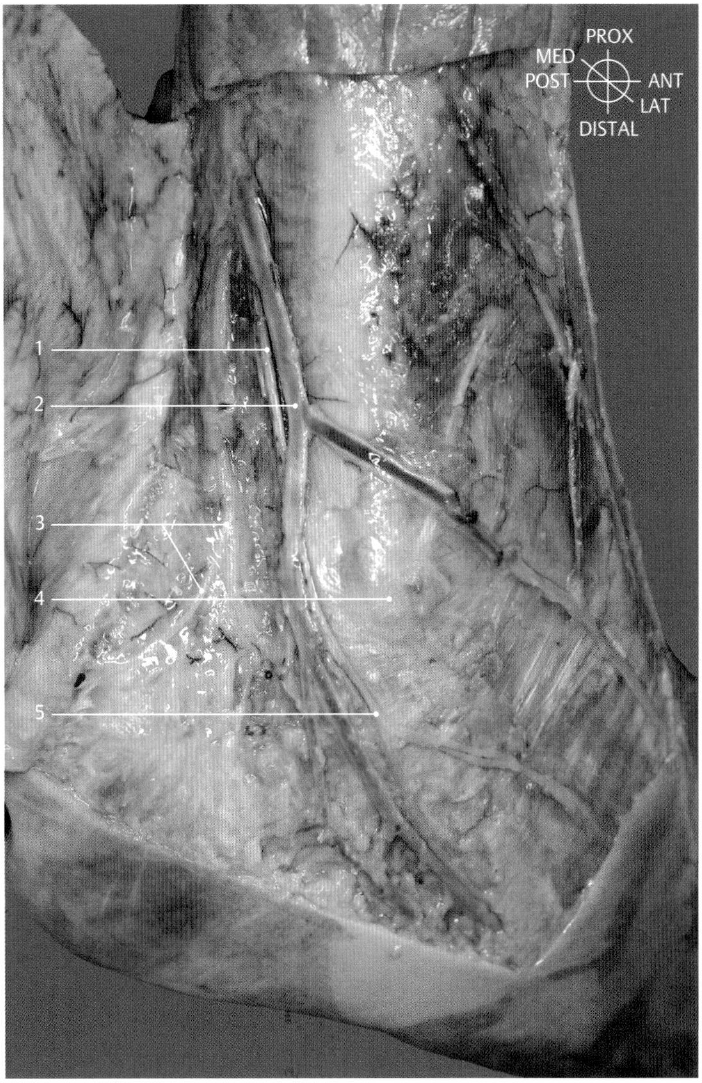

Fig. 6.27 Posterolateral view of a right ankle to show the structures at risk during placement of a posterolateral portal.

1 Sural nerve
2 Lesser saphenous vein
3 Lateral calcaneal branches (sural nerve)
4 Fibula
5 Lateral dorsal cutaneous nerve (sural nerve)

Posteromedial Portal

For this portal the structures at risk are (from lateral to medial) the flexor hallucis longus, the flexor digitorum longus muscle tendons, and the tibialis posterior neurovascular bundle (**Fig. 6.28**).

Figs. 6.29–6.31 show the deep anatomy of the posterior ankle. The goal is to show the limits of the posterior arthroscopic working space, the osseous structures, tendons, and ligaments.

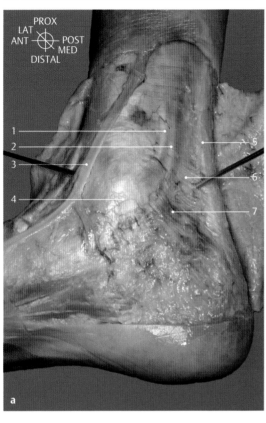

Fig. 6.28 (a–c) Posteromedial views of a right ankle show the medial structures and their relation with the posteromedial portal.

1 Tibialis posterior muscle tendon
2 Flexor digitorum longus muscle tendon
3 Great saphenous vein
4 Medial malleolus
5 Calcaneus tendon
6 Neurovascular bundle
7 Flexor retinaculum

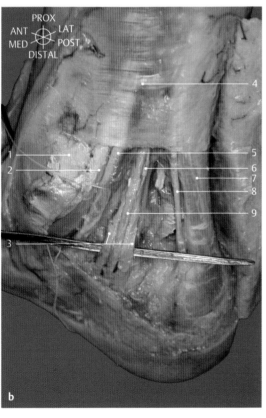

(b) Posteromedial view of a right ankle shows the medial structures and their relation with the posteromedial portal.

1 Medial malleolus
2 Tibialis posterior muscle tendon
3 Lateral and medial branches of the tibialis nerve
4 Flexor retinaculum
5 Flexor digitorum longus muscle tendon
6 Tibialis nerve
7 Calcaneus tendon
8 Plantaris tendon
9 Tibialis posterior artery

(Continued)

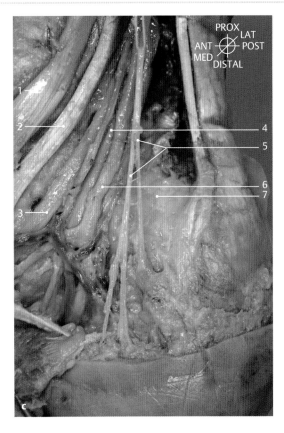

Fig. 6.28   (*continued*)
(c) Posteromedial view of a right ankle shows the medial structures and their relation with the posteromedial portal.

1 Tibialis posterior muscle tendon
2 Flexor digitorum longus muscle tendon
3 Medial plantaris nerve
4 Lateral plantaris nerve
5 Medial branches (calcaneal nerve)
6 Tibialis posterior artery
7 Calcaneus

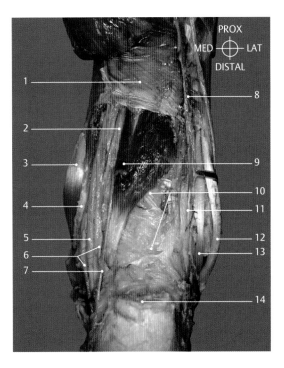

Fig. 6.29   Posterior view of a right ankle showing the medial and lateral structures. The calcaneus tendon is sectioned and moved proximally to see the posterior arthroscopic working area; the medial limit is marked by the flexor hallucis longus muscle tendon. The image shows why it is important to respect this limit due to the great risk of a neurovascular lesion.

1 Flexor retinaculum
2 Tibial nerve
3 Tibialis posterior muscle tendon
4 Flexor digitorum longus muscle tendon
5 Tibialis posterior artery
6 Tibialis posterior veins
7 Medial calcaneal branches of tibial nerve
8 Lesser saphenous vein
9 Flexor hallucis longus muscle
10 Retrocalcaneal fat pad
11 Sural nerve
12 Fibularis longus muscle tendon
13 Fibularis brevis muscle tendon
14 Calcaneal tendon (cut)

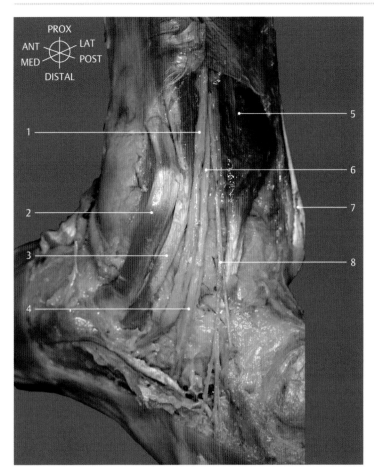

Fig. 6.30 Posteromedial view of the posterior arthroscopic working area in a right ankle.

1 Posterior tibial artery
2 Tibialis posterior muscle tendon
3 Flexor digitorum longus muscle tendon
4 Lateral plantaris nerve
5 Flexor hallucis longus muscle
6 Tibial nerve
7 Fibularis longus and brevis tendons
8 Medial calcaneal branches (tibial nerve)

181

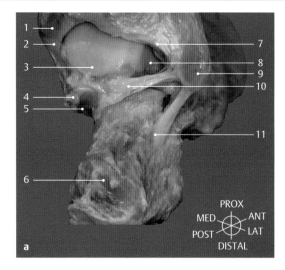 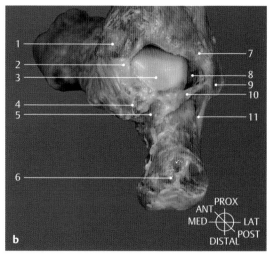

Fig. 6.31 **(a, b)** Posterior views of a right ankle showing the osseous structures and ligaments evaluated in a posterior arthroscopy of the ankle. The sulcus of the flexor hallucis longus muscle tendon (medial limit) and the posterolateral recess (lateral limit) are shown.

1 Medial malleolus, 2 Posterior tibiotalar part of deltoid ligament, 3 Talus, 4 Sustentaculum tali, 5 Sulcus tendinis flexor hallucis longus muscle, 6 Calcaneus, 7 Posterior tibiofibular ligament, 8 Lateral malleolar fossa, sulcus malleolaris, 9 Lateral malleolus, 10 Posterior talofibular ligament, 11 Calcaneofibular ligament

6.3.6 Arthroscopic Examination of the Ankle via the Posterolateral Portal

The posterolateral portal (the "safe" portal) is established at the level of the posterior articular line (1–1.5 cm proximal to the distal tip of the fibula), just lateral to the edge of the calcaneus tendon. The direction of the arthroscope is in line with the second metatarsal bone. This position is unchanged until the posteromedial portal is established. The posteromedial portal is an instrumentation portal. It is the most dangerous portal because of the possible neurovascular complications. To avoid these complications the shaver tip should always contact the arthroscopic cannula when opening the posterior working space of the ankle. The shaver slides down the arthroscope moving toward the tip, opening the posterior space to identify the tibiotalar articular joint and the medial limit that is the flexor hallucis longus tendon (**Fig. 6.32**).

The suggested sequence for an arthroscopic examination of the posterior ankle is shown in **Figs. 6.33–6.38**. The use of invasive distraction is optional.

1. Initial arthroscopic view (**Fig. 6.33**)

2. Arthroscopic view of the flexor hallucis longus muscle tendon (**Fig. 6.34**)

3. Arthroscopic view of the tibiotalar joint (**Figs. 6.35** and **6.36**)

4. Arthroscopic view of the subtalar joint (**Fig. 6.37**)

5. Anatomical–arthroscopic relation of the flexor hallucis longus tendon and the posterior tibial nerve (**Fig. 6.38**)

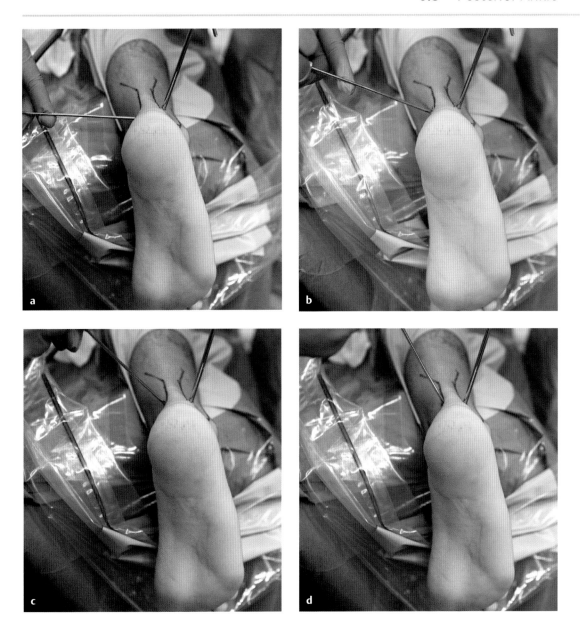

Fig. 6.32   (a–d) Posterolateral and posteromedial portal placements in a right ankle.

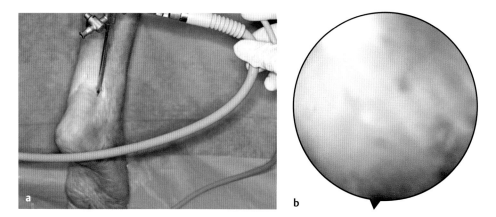

Fig. 6.33 **(a)** Posterior view of a right (cadaveric) ankle with the arthroscope in the posterolateral portal and the corresponding initial arthroscopic view. The soft tissue in front of the posterior working space of the ankle is shown in the arthroscopic view. This space must be opened up by resecting the corresponding tissue. **(b)** Arthroscopic view.

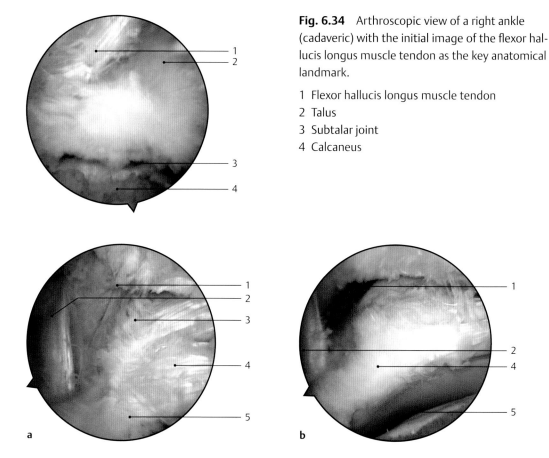

Fig. 6.34 Arthroscopic view of a right ankle (cadaveric) with the initial image of the flexor hallucis longus muscle tendon as the key anatomical landmark.

1 Flexor hallucis longus muscle tendon
2 Talus
3 Subtalar joint
4 Calcaneus

Fig. 6.35 **(a, b)** Arthroscopic views of a right ankle (cadaveric) via the posterolateral portal. The posterior tibiotalar joint capsule must be opened to get access to this joint.

1 Tibiotalar joint—medial recess, 2 Flexor hallucis longus muscle tendon, 3 Posterior tibiotalar joint capsule (posterior intermalleolar ligament (resected)), 4 Posterior talofibular ligament, 5 Subtalar joint

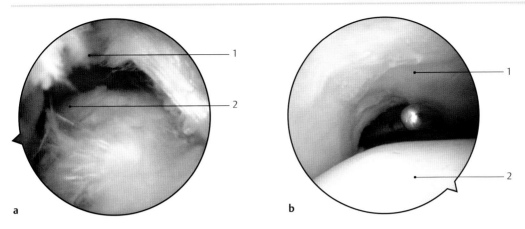

Fig. 6.36 **(a, b)** Arthroscopic views of a right (cadaveric) ankle; the tibiotalar joint is evaluated using invasive distraction. The probe is in the anteromedial portal.

1 Distal articular surface of the tibia, 2 Talus

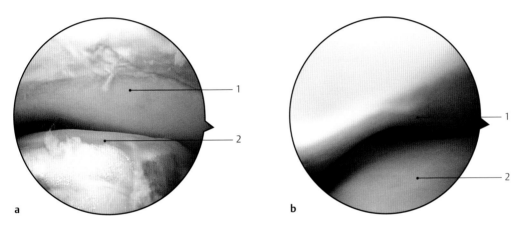

Fig. 6.37 **(a, b)** Right (cadaveric) ankle distracted for an arthroscopic subtalar joint evaluation.

1 Subtalar articular surface of the talus, 2 Subtalar articular surface of the calcaneus

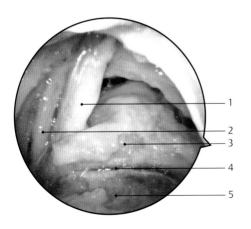

Fig. 6.38 Arthroscopic view of a right (cadaveric) ankle that shows the close relation between the flexor hallucis longus muscle tendon and the tibial nerve.

1 Flexor hallucis longus muscle tendon
2 Tibial nerve
3 Talus
4 Subtalar joint
5 Calcaneus

185

6.3.7 Additional Aspects of the Anterior and Posterior Anatomy of the Ankle

These cuts allow a further understanding of the ankle joint anatomy for a safer arthroscopic technique, as discussed previously (**Figs. 6.39–6.41**).

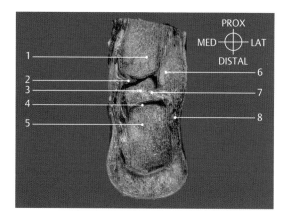

Fig. 6.39   Coronal cut.
1 Tibia
2 Tibiotalar joint (synovial fold)
3 Talus
4 Subtalar joint
5 Calcaneus
6 Fibula
7 Posterior talofibular ligament
8 Fibularis brevis and longus muscle tendons

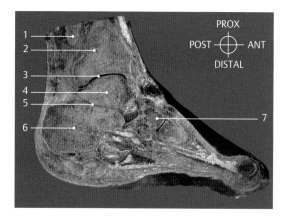

Fig. 6.40   Sagittal cut.
1 Fibula
2 Tibia
3 Tibiotalar joint
4 Talus
5 Subtalar joint
6 Calcaneus
7 Navicular

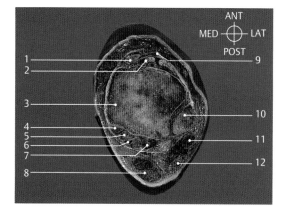

Fig. 6.41   Transverse cut.
1 Tibialis anterior tendon
2 Anterior tibial artery/deep peroneal nerve
3 Tibia
4 Tibialis posterior muscle tendon
5 Flexor digitorum longus muscle tendon
6 Posterior tibial artery, vein, nerve
7 Flexor hallucis longus muscle tendon
8 Calcaneus tendon
9 Extensor digitorum longus muscle tendon
10 Fibula
11 Peroneus brevis/longus tendons
12 Sural nerve and small saphenous vein

Index

Page numbers in *italics* refer to illustrations

187